Contents

Foreword

In the last 15 years the bookshelves have filled with publications about sexual abuse. There are personal accounts, self-help manuals, how-to texts written from different theoretical perspectives and in a variety of formats, research findings and academic tomes. It could be argued that by now we must have something for everyone, but this is not the case. *Counselling a Survivor of Child Sexual Abuse: a person-centred dialogue* brings a unique and powerful insight into the qualitative process that engages both client and counsellor in a person-centred setting. Richard Bryant-Jefferies has eloquently and comprehensively conveyed the conditions of relating that are the very essence of person-centred work.

In his introduction, the author provides a useful guide to the impact of sexual abuse which, by way of the references, could be used as a springboard into further reading. Unlike many other books on this topic we are not plunged in at the deep end; instead by explaining the background and reviewing the case we are introduced to the characters and the scene is set.

The presentation style will seem familiar to many – those who have undertaken person-centred training or carried out qualitative counselling research will recognise the similarity to transcripts of audio-taped sessions. Throughout the dialogue, boxes are placed in the text which draw out points of learning, educate and inform the reader or pose questions and prompt reflection. This presentation particularly lends itself to highlighting pertinent issues from a flowing and emerging process that typifies person-centred work. Just as the symbols on a map provide information about the terrain we might encounter on a journey, so these asides from the dialogue impart knowledge which helps the reader understand the territory through which our two companions are travelling.

The author sensitively covers key issues faced by survivors of abuse – the fear of dissociation, coming to terms with recovered memories, working with feelings of blame, grief and anger. He highlights dilemmas faced by counsellors such as the threat of premature ending, staying with and containing a client in dissociative states, dealing with crises, managing breaks and staying in the client's frame. The picture is completed by the inclusion of the supervisory dialogue which, just like the review at the beginning, places the process in its rightful setting, creating an authentic feel to the book as well as touching on topics such as parallel process and on providing conditions of acceptance of the counsellor's own process.

This is a book that succeeds in a number of ways. For a beginner it is full of knowledge and wisdom that gives a broad view of the issues. For someone experienced in this field the book highlights points for reflection and discussion on the dilemmas of counselling survivors of child sexual abuse in general and the rigours demanded of person-centred practitioners in particular. Richard Bryant-Jefferies has also succeeded in writing a book that is a valuable teaching aid. At the end of each chapter there are a number of points for discussion which provide excellent learning points to prompt discussion and encourage further exploration of themes raised at each stage. In many training environments this would be a valuable addition to the reading list.

Linda Hughes Dip Psych & Couns
May 2003

Linda Hughes is a psychotherapist and a founding director of The Kernos Centre in Sudbury, Suffolk. Her main area of expertise is in working with people who have experienced trauma and abuse in childhood, people with eating disorders and those who self-injure. She has a wealth of clinical experience as well as expertise in teaching and training. In 1994, she established the first university accredited course in the UK to train healthcare professionals in working with survivors of childhood abuse. She joined the clinical team at Lapis in Colchester in 1993 and was clinical administrator of the counselling service until 1999. At that time she became a Fellow at the University of Essex, where she created and taught a certificate course in working with abuse. Linda trained with the Client-Centred Approach Institute International and now practises as a humanistic therapist, being a fully accredited member of the Association of Humanistic Psychology Practitioners.

Foreword

One of the paradoxical qualities of dissociation, in my experience, is the fact that even quite experienced therapists can have this happen right in front of their eyes and manage not to see it. A therapist can pass by a strangely puzzling moment that comes and goes in an otherwise coherent client story and forget that it happened. Or, she can convince herself that the client really meant to say something very ordinary, when in reality the client has managed to give some small indication of the desperation and strangeness of his or her inner experiences after great personal struggle.

I have found that when therapists do not manage to create an open and safe space for clients' first attempts to speak from dissociative aspects of their experience, clients often cooperate by keeping drastically abusive early experiences completely separate from the therapy process. After all, clients are not sure that they can survive the memory of these experiences themselves and they are not sure that any other human being could ever understand them. The tragic result of this, in my experience, is that their therapists only become aware of the outer edges of dissociative experiences when they emerge in more external, out-of-control manifestations such as suicide attempts, cutting, anxiety attacks, physical collapse or self-destructive use of drugs and alcohol.

Therapist attunement to this process makes all the difference. For a client-centered therapist, this involves an exceedingly delicate balance between taking the client's words at face value and sensing times when the client is engaged in a struggle between parts of them that want to say more and other parts that prohibit them from speaking. If the therapist is not right with the client at these moments, clients are very likely to conclude that the therapist is unable to handle what they are trying to say and to move back to safer subjects or more indirect ways of speaking. In my own attempts to speak and write about dissociated process I have always felt frustrated at my limitations in expressing how this delicate balance plays out in actual client-centered therapy work. On the one hand, successful client-centered work with dissociation is the most non-directive and moment-to-moment empathic work imaginable. On the other hand, there is a significant role played by the therapist's understanding of how dissociation works and what might be surfacing in the client. Faced with my own limitations in expressing this balance, I have had to hope that, given some preliminary knowledge, young counselors and therapists would discover it for themselves when dissociated process emerged in their own practice.

Given all of this, I am amazed at the degree to which Richard Bryant-Jefferies has been able to catch the feel of an actual therapy relationship involving the recovery of dissociated trauma memories in the relationship between 'Laura' and 'Jennifer' as portrayed in this book. Many of the passages in this fictional account gave me goose bumps reading them. I thought, 'Yes, this is exactly what those moments of therapy feel like to me when clients first venture into trying to express dissociative experiences'. I think that this moment-to-moment account of a therapy relationship is likely to be invaluable to therapists learning to work with this sort of material as it emerges with their own clients.

And, I think that the openness of the approach that Richard Bryant-Jefferies takes to this account is likely to be particularly valuable to readers. While this is an account of a very successful, and to me very realistic-seeming, therapy relationship, the author is careful to explain that he is not trying to portray a perfect client, a perfect therapist or a perfect supervisor. This leaves the reader free to ask him- or herself, 'How would I have responded in that situation?', or, 'Do I think that the therapist or supervisor was really keeping Rogers' core conditions at that moment?' This account makes clear the degree to which the person-centered relationship involves a very personal, very individual process rather than any set of pre-set meanings or directives.

Actual clients experiencing dissociation are, of course, very different from each other. Many clients take longer than the client described in this book as they approach and work through severe incest memories; some are unable to persevere in facing these experiences at all. Some, like this client, have lived seemingly high functioning lives for a long time. Others have had lives of obvious chaos and mental breakdown. Many of the particular ways that dissociated parts manifest themselves are unique to the individual client. Still, despite all of these differences, there is something about the feel of dissociated experiences that seems quite similar to me between clients. And, for me, there is something about the courage of clients who struggle to reclaim lost parts of their experience that is incredibly moving.

My strongest hope is that readers of this current book will find a similar respect for, and interest in, clients struggling with dissociated experiences and find themselves wanting to open themselves up to this sort of work in their own counseling and therapy practices.

Margaret S Warner PhD
Professor, Illinois School of Professional Psychology, Chicago Campus
May 2003

Margaret S Warner is a client-centered teacher and theorist who has written extensively about the value of client-centered therapy in working with clients who face more serious psychological disorders, and on client-centered theory as it relates to other disciplines in clinical psychology and the behavioral sciences.

She trained in client-centered therapy at the Chicago Counseling Center, an offshoot of Carl Rogers' original Center at the University of Chicago. She has a doctorate in Behavioral Sciences from the University of Chicago, and is currently a Professor at the Illinois School of Professional Psychology, Chicago Campus.

She was one of the organizers of Chicago 2000: The Fifth International Conference on Client-Centered and Experiential Psychotherapy and is currently working to develop a Minor and Certificate Program in Client-Centered and Experiential Psychology at the Illinois School.

About the author

Richard Bryant-Jefferies qualified as a person-centred counsellor/therapist in 1994 and remains passionate about the application and effectiveness of this approach. Since early 1995 Richard has worked at a community drug and alcohol service in Surrey. As well as offering counselling within this specialist arena, he also supervises counsellors who work with people with drug and alcohol problems, works himself as a general counsellor in a GP surgery and offers general counselling supervision, including supervision of counsellors working with young people. He also offers training in 'Alcohol Awareness and Response' (www.bryant-jefferies.freeserve.co.uk) for anyone working with people who have alcohol problems.

He has worked with a number of people who have used alcohol and other substances to cope with the traumatic effects of child sexual abuse and is concerned that in a society where health services emphasise physical and mental health, often those with traumatised emotions can struggle to receive the service they require. He is also aware of how often clients with traumatically abusive experience in their past find it difficult to receive therapeutic support whilst they continue to use a substance, and yet they are unable to stop or control their use because of the feelings of distress that overwhelm them. He is convinced, from his own experience, that you can work with people therapeutically who are still using substances.

Richard had his first book on a counselling theme published in 2001, *Counselling the Person Beyond the Alcohol Problem* (Jessica Kingsley Publishers), providing theoretical yet practical insights into the application of the person-centred approach within the context of the 'cycle of change' model that has been widely adopted to describe the process of change in the field of addiction. Since then he has been writing for the *Living Therapy* series (Radcliffe Medical Press), producing an on-going series of person-centred dialogues: *Problem Drinking, Time Limited Therapy in Primary Care, Counselling a Recovering Drug User, Counselling Young People* and *Counselling for Progressive Disability*. The aim of the series is to bring the reader a direct experience of the counselling process, an exposure to the thoughts and feelings of both client and counsellor as they encounter each other on the therapeutic journey, and an insight into the value and importance of supervision.

Richard is keen to bring the experience of the therapeutic process, from the standpoint and application of the person-centred approach, to a wider audience.

He is convinced that the principles and attitudinal values of this approach and the emphasis it places on the therapeutic relationship are key to helping people create greater authenticity both in themselves and in their lives, leading to a fuller and more satisfying human experience.

Acknowledgements

I would like to acknowledge and thank all the people who have offered me support and encouragement in writing this book. In particular, Jan Hawkins for sharing her insight and experience both prior to me starting the writing, and on reading through the final draft of the text. Jan specialises in working with people who are survivors of childhood abuse and offers training in this area. I have very much valued her contribution.

I also wish to thank David Voyle, a colleague and a counsellor like myself specialising in working with people with alcohol problems, who, over recent years, has contributed in a major way to my thinking on this topic, and particularly in relation to the numbers of clients with alcohol problems in adulthood who have been targets for sexual abuse during their childhood.

Once again, I wish to thank Maggie Pettifer, series editor, for her continued enthusiasm and encouragement, and Radcliffe Medical Press for their belief in this fictitious dialogue approach as a way of helping people better understand the process and demands of person-centred counselling, and its application to particular difficulties and within different counselling settings.

Introduction

This latest book in the *Living Therapy* series has been written with the express intention of providing the reader with insight into the living experience of working with a client who is a survivor of child sexual abuse. The counsellor works from the person-centred model and, as with previous books in this series, *Problem Drinking: a person-centred dialogue* (Bryant-Jefferies, 2003) and *Time Limited Therapy in Primary Care: a person-centred dialogue* (Bryant-Jefferies, 2003), the actual dialogue and the characters involved are all fictitious. It is not intended that the counsellor or the supervisor be portrayed as perfect in their work, that would be unrealistic and would therefore be incongruent to the aim of this book, which is to offer a realistic experience. The counsellor takes the work he or she is doing with their client to regular supervision, and these sessions are also included. They provide an added dimension to the work being undertaken and offer the reader an appreciation of the use of supervision as both a personal and professional discipline to ensure healthy and safe practice both for the welfare of the client and the counsellor.

Points for discussion are included at the end of each chapter, offering an opportunity for the book to be utilised within a training environment as well as providing the reader with specific themes on which to reflect further.

The book is not written in order to provide a definitive example of person-centred counselling. It does, however, provide insight into ways in which the approach can have application when working with this client group.

Whether to use the term 'child' or 'childhood' in referring to the sexual abuse has been something I have reflected on and discussed with others, meeting with mixed responses. It is a child that is sexually abused and traumatically affected. The sexual abuse is perpetrated within the developmental context of childhood experiencing. I have therefore found myself using both 'child sexual abuse' and 'childhood sexual abuse' in different places.

The abbreviation CSA, often used to indicate child sexual abuse, is not used. I feel that the abbreviation can divert the reader from the reality of what is being referred to and described. It can sanitise, be spoken or read too quickly without allowing time for the real words that they represent to strike a chord and evoke a reaction. Authenticity demands that we say it as it is.

This book does contain some necessary sexually explicit references, required to ensure realism. However, it is written with the aim of evoking from the reader personal feelings, thoughts and reactions to help inform practice. To work with clients who are experiencing extreme psychological reactions to sexual, physical and emotional trauma requires the counsellor to know themselves and to have largely resolved their own issues concerning the area being dealt with. I say largely resolved because I am not convinced that issues are necessarily or always totally resolved. What is vital, however, is that the counsellor has done the personal development work to enable them to be clear as to their own attitudes and where they originate, and that they are open to question their reactions to what is presented to them by their clients.

I do not believe there are specific answers or treatments for these kinds of traumatic experience. Every survivor of child sexual abuse needs to come to terms with it in their own way, and the person-centred counsellor or therapist believes that the survivor has within themselves the resources for this, they simply need an appropriate and therapeutic relational environment. In a world where we seem to be beset by a trend towards 'manualising treatment modalities' the person-centred approach stands and says NO, that is not the way forward. Listen to the client, and let them know what you have heard as accurately as you can. Listen to the client and accept the reality of their inner world, unconditionally. Listen to the client and trust their capacity to discover their own inner wisdom and resources.

In writing this book, I had no idea from chapter to chapter, page to page, even word to word, what would happen next. It simply evolved, with the characters – Jennifer, Laura and Malcolm – developing as the narrative unfolded. This may sound weird, but I want to thank them for coming into my life, for in writing this book I have learned a great deal, both about the subject and about myself. Yes, as the writer, I also am and was affected by what has been written. I am grateful for that.

At the end of the book I have included some final thoughts. They evolved through my experience of writing this book. I know I am changed as a result of this process, and I value this. If I could not have felt affected by what I was writing then I would have no reason to expect others to be touched or moved themselves. More than anything else, I have wanted to try to offer the reader an opportunity to engage with themselves more fully and openly as they enter into the world of person-centred counselling and supervision in the context of working with a survivor of child sexual abuse.

Child sexual abuse

Child sexual abuse can still seem a taboo area for some, and it has been noted that 'the counselling of adult survivors of childhood sexual abuse has long been hindered by the denial of the phenomenon' (Draucker, 1992, p. 3). The reality is that child sexual abuse is a major cause of many of the physical, emotional, mental and psychological problems that are brought by people into counselling.

Neither the phenomenon nor the psychological impact were truly recognised as essentially problematic until the French neurologist Jean-Martin Charcot began to study hysteria during the latter part of the nineteenth century, attracting the attention of many other notable pioneers in the fields of psychiatry and neurology. Then later, as Janet, Freud and Breuer began to spend time listening to and documenting their clients describing their experiences of sexual violence and exploitation, came the idea that hysteria was in fact a symptom of traumatic experiencing. Freud, in particular, found himself driven, perhaps by his own curiosity, into deeper empathic listening to his female patients as they described to him histories of sexual abuse, rape and incestuous relationships. In 1896 he produced a report on a series of case studies in which he made the claim: 'I therefore put forward the thesis that at the bottom of every case of hysteria there are *one or more occurrences of premature sexual experience*, occurrences which belong to the earliest years of childhood . . .' (Freud, 1896).

Nevertheless, Freud was later to repudiate his ideas. Having discovered that hysteria was so common among women he realised that if his theory was correct then what he termed as ' "perverted acts against children" were endemic, not only among the proletariat in Paris, where he had first studied hysteria, but also among the respectable bourgeois families of Vienna, where he had established his practice' (Herman, 1994, p. 14). Referring to Freud's notes, papers and letters, Herman goes on to indicate that this would have been considered unacceptable and beyond credibility (Bonaparte *et al.*, 1954). The idea of sexual abuse as a primary cause of hysteria became discredited, with Freud himself taking the view that it was in fact due to fantasy. Scientific interest on the topic collapsed.

Later, during the 1940s, a series of studies were undertaken, including the Kinsey *et al.* study of 1953, referred to by Draucker (1992, p. 4). These studies found that 20–30% of female respondents reported childhood sexual experiences with a male, between 4 and 12% reported sexual experience with a relative, and 1% reported sexual experience with a father or stepfather. Later still, with the rise of the feminist movement, further scientific studies were inspired, leading to a greater awakening to the widespread reality of child sexual abuse.

Louise Armstrong, cited as being 'one of the first feminist authors to expose father–daughter sexual abuse' (Bagley and King, 1990, p. 47), is quoted as follows in describing her perspective on the attitude of the perpetrator and its effect on the victim: 'Repeated sexual abuse of a child by a needed and trusted parent or step-parent is the most purely gratuitous form of abuse there is. It requires thought. It does not arise out of anything as uncontrollable as rage . . . It does not stem from physical addiction. Rather, it arises out of an assumed prerogative, super-structured with rationale, protected by traditions of silence, and, even more than in rape, an assurance of the object's continuing fear, shame, powerlessness and, therefore, silent acquiescence' (Armstrong, 1978, p. 277).

Prevalence studies frequently reveal wide ranges which are likely to be linked to the varying definitions of sexual abuse, in particular as to whether non-contact sexual abuse is included in the surveys. For instance, a survey of 930 women in San Fransisco (Russell, 1983, 1986) reported 54% as having had at least one experience of child sexual abuse prior to the age of 18 where the survey included both intra- and extra-familial perpetrators and both contact and non-contact acts of sexual abuse. This contrasts with an overview of child sexual abuse prevalence studies that found the incidence ranging from 6–62% among females and 3–31% among males (Peters *et al.*, 1986).

Much has been written concerning the longer-term effects of the experience of sexual abuse in childhood. Emotional effects include depression, low self-esteem, guilt, shame, anxiety, anger and obsessive/compulsive disorders (Sanderson, 1990), together with problems with interpersonal relationships, sexual dysfunction, suicidal states and generally self-destructive behaviours, including substance misuse. Draucker (1992) provides an informative summary of the characteristic longer-term effects of child sexual abuse.

Substance use/misuse can help the survivor to block memories and internal discomfort that may, or may not, be reaching conscious awareness. Spak *et al.* (1997, p. 273) reported that child sexual abuse was the strongest predictor for the later development of alcohol abuse, together with a history of psychiatric problems. They also added that sexual abuse prior to age 13 exacerbated presenting symptoms. This was supported by Swett *et al.* (1991, p. 57), whose research indicated that physical or sexual abuse prior to the age of 18 may be associated with a higher consumption of alcohol compared to those who had not experienced sexual abuse in childhood.

Yet statistics can only take us so far in our understanding and preparation to work with survivors of child sexual abuse. Working with a survivor of child sexual abuse is challenging to the therapist. Sanderson (1990) makes the point that whilst a counsellor may prepare themselves for the nature and content of a session when working with a survivor by reading first-hand accounts, 'it is not the same as facing a survivor displaying so much anguish, fear and distress'. She also wisely argues that, 'it is essential for the counsellor to not only have a satisfactory support network and supervision, but also to have alternative activities in which to relax and regenerate depleted resources of energy and emotion to prevent therapist burn-out' (Sanderson, 1990, p. 227).

For the client for whom the experience of child sexual abuse has become a repressed memory, it is highly likely that this needs to emerge into consciousness as part of the therapeutic process. This can, and generally is, extremely traumatic for the client, but the release of feelings and the process of creating an understanding of what has occurred and the effect it has had on later life, helps the client to reintegrate and achieve some relief from traumatic symptomology, or at least offers greater scope for self-management. Such a process may also result in some degree of relief from the symptoms of post-traumatic effects (Herman and Schatzow, 1987).

The person-centred counsellor or therapist will not be introducing the possibility of child sexual abuse whatever the symptomology presented by the client, but will allow the client to explore what is present for them within their own experience, and the associated meanings that they have developed. The search for meaning has been recognised as an important feature of coping with traumatic experience. Taylor (1983, p. 1161) defines meaning as 'an effort to understand the event: why it happened and what impact it had'. The person-centred counsellor trusts the working of the actualising tendency to bring to the client's attention experiences and memories when the time is right for them to be addressed, which is often when the client's structure of self can no longer maintain concealment of them from normal waking consciousness. This can also occur when alcohol consumption, or any tranquillising medication or substance, is reduced.

The person-centred therapist will be seeking to establish psychological contact with the client, ensuring that the core therapeutic conditions of empathy, congruence and unconditional positive regard are maintained, communicated and received by the client. 'The quality of a therapeutic relationship and the outcome of treatment are both strongly influenced by the level of empathic understanding exhibited by the therapist and perceived by the client' (Goldstein, 1980).

Yet the client may well be fragmented within their self-structure, providing many aspects of themselves, each equally in need of being heard and warmly accepted. Margaret Warner has formulated her own theory on the topic of 'dissociative states and processes' within the person that develop in response to traumatic experiencing (Warner, 1998, 2000). She describes them in the following way: ' "Dissociated" process is a style of process in which aspects of the person's experience are separated into "parts" – personified clusters of experience which may be partially or totally unaware of each other's presence. These parts have trance-like qualities, allowing the person to alter perceptions, to alter physiological states and to hold contradictory beliefs without discomfort. Such parts seem to have been created in early childhood as a way to keep the person from being overwhelmed by experiences of incest or other abuse' (Warner, 2000, p. 145).

The person-centred counsellor will be challenged by such dissociative states and processes within the person of the client. Indeed, they could easily be mistaken for psychotic states, and care needs to be taken on this point. Clients with what has become known as dissociative identity disorder (DID) should not be labelled 'mentally ill'. They have experienced traumatic events in their early lives and they need to experience a healing relationship to help them re-integrate their often profoundly individual and separate parts.

Some dissociated parts may be more present than others, some may struggle to be heard, e.g. the voice of the abused child who has somehow to confront other dissociated parts that conspire to maintain silence on the abuse that occurred. All parts require the empathic understanding and warm acceptance of the authentic counsellor. Each has developed and has a place within the client's structure of self, contributing to the uniqueness of that person. As Margaret Warner continues in her description: 'They may influence behaviour while remaining out of the person's consciousness as "others" whose images and voices have an impact on the person. Or, they may emerge as temporarily dominant personalities who take control of the person's consciousness for a period of time' (Warner, 2000, p. 145).

Within the dialogue of this book are further references to this developing area of person-centred theory as it has particular application to working with clients who are survivors of sexual abuse in their childhood.

The following pages are written to take you into an experience, an opportunity to gain a deeper understanding and appreciation of the client who is a survivor, of the therapist who is working with the client, of the therapeutic process that develops between them, of the role of the counsellor's supervisor and, of course, of yourself as you react and associate your own meanings to the experiences contained in this book.

> *Don't give up. That's the best thing I could tell somebody who just remembered she was a survivor. There are people who have lived through it, and as trite and stupid as it sounds to you right now, you will not be in so much pain later. If you made it this far, you've got some pretty good stuff in you. Don't give up on yourself.*
>
> Catherine, 35-year-old survivor (Bass and Davis, 1993)

The person-centred approach

The person-centred approach (PCA) was formulated by Carl Rogers, and references are made to his ideas within the text of this book. However, it will be helpful for readers who are unfamiliar with this way of working to have an appreciation of its theoretical base.

Rogers proposed that certain conditions, when present within a therapeutic relationship, would enable the client to develop towards what he termed 'fuller functionality'. Over a number of years he refined these ideas, which he defined as 'the necessary and sufficient conditions for constructive personality change'. He described these in papers in the late 1950s (Rogers, 1957, p. 96):

1 Two persons are in psychological contact.
2 The first, whom we shall term the client, is in a state of incongruence, being vulnerable or anxious.
3 The second person, whom we shall term the therapist, is congruent or integrated in the relationship.
4 The therapist experiences unconditional positive regard for the client.
5 The therapist experiences an empathic understanding of the client's internal frame of reference and endeavours to communicate this experience to the client.
6 The communication to the client of the therapist's empathic understanding and unconditional positive regard is to a minimal degree achieved.

Rogers defined empathy as meaning 'entering the private perceptual world of the other ... being sensitive, moment by moment, to the changing felt meanings which flow in this other person ... It means sensing meanings of which he or she is scarcely aware, but not trying to uncover totally unconscious feelings' (Rogers, 1980, p. 142). It is a very delicate process, and it provides, I believe, a foundation block. The counsellor's role is primarily to establish empathic rapport and to communicate empathic understanding to the client.

Within this relationship the counsellor seeks to maintain an attitude of unconditional positive regard towards the client and all that they disclose. This is not 'agreeing with', it is simply warm acceptance. Rogers wrote, 'when the therapist is experiencing a positive, acceptant attitude towards whatever the client *is* at that moment, therapeutic movement or change is more likely to occur' (Rogers, 1980, p. 116). Mearns and Thorne suggest that 'unconditional positive regard is the label given to the fundamental attitude of the person-centred counsellor towards her client. The counsellor who holds this attitude deeply values the humanity of her client and is not deflected in that valuing by any particular client behaviours. The attitude manifests itself in the counsellor's consistent acceptance of and enduring warmth towards her client' (Mearns and Thorne, 1988, p. 59).

Last, but by no means least, is the state of being that Rogers referred to as congruence, but which has also been described in terms of 'realness', 'transparency', 'genuineness', 'authenticity'. Indeed, Rogers wrote that '... genuineness, realness or congruence ... this means that the therapist is openly being the feelings and attitudes that are flowing within at the moment ... the term transparent catches the flavour of this condition'. Putting this into the therapeutic setting, we can say that 'congruence is the state of being of the counsellor when her outward responses to her client consistently match the inner feelings and sensations which she has in relation to her client' (Mearns and Thorne, 1999, p. 84).

I would suggest that any congruent expression by the counsellor of their feelings or reactions has to emerge through the process of being in therapeutic relationship with the client. It is a disciplined response and not an open door to endless self-disclosure. Congruent expression is perhaps most appropriate and therapeutically valuable where it is informed by the existence of an empathic understanding of the client's inner world, and is offered in a climate of a genuine warm acceptance towards the client.

PCA regards the relationship that we have with our clients, and the attitude that we hold within that relationship, to be key factors. In my experience, many adult psychological difficulties develop out of life experiences that involve problematic, conditional or abusive relational experiences. This can be centred in childhood or later in life. What is important is that the individual is left, through relationships that have a negative conditioning effect, with a distorted perception of themselves and their potential as a person. I see many people who have learned from childhood experience beliefs such as 'I can never be good enough to be praised for what I have achieved; I never match my parents' expectations' or 'No one was ever there for me when I was hurting; perhaps I am unlovable'. The result is a loss of a positive sense of self, and the individual adapts to maintain the newly learned concept of self. This is then lived out, possibly throughout life, with the person seeking to satisfy what they have come to believe about themselves: being unable to achieve, feeling unable to be loved, though perhaps in both cases maintaining a constant desperation to receive what they never had. Yet, perversely, they may then sabotage any possibility of gaining what they want in order to maintain the negatively conditioned sense of self.

It is my belief that by offering someone a non-judgemental, warm, accepting and authentic relationship, the person can grow into a fresh sense of self in which their potential as a person can become more fulfilled. Such an experience fosters an opportunity for the client to redefine themselves as they experience the presence of the therapist's congruence, empathy and unconditional positive regard. This process can take time. Often the personality change that is required to sustain a shift away from what have been termed 'conditions of worth' requires a lengthy period of therapeutic work, bearing in mind that the person may be struggling to unravel a sense of self that has been developed, sustained and reinforced for many decades of life.

The term 'conditions of worth' applies to the conditioning that is frequently present in childhood, and at other times in life, when a person experiences that their worth is conditional on their doing something, or behaving, in a certain way. This is usually to satisfy someone else's needs, and can be contrary to the client's own sense of what would be a satisfying experience. The values of others become a feature of the individual's structure of self. The person moves away from being true to themselves, learning instead to remain 'true' to their conditioned sense of worth. This state of being in the client is challenged by the person-centred therapist offering them unconditional positive regard and warm acceptance. Such a therapist, by genuinely offering these therapeutic attitudes, provides the client with an opportunity to be exposed to what may be a new experience or one that in the past they have dismissed, preferring to stay with that which matches and therefore reinforces their conditioned sense of worth and sense of self. Unconditional positive regard and warm acceptance offered consistently over time can, and does, enable clients to begin to question their beliefs about themselves and to begin to build into their structure of self the capacity to see and experience themselves as being of value for who they are. It enables them to liberate themselves from the constraints of patterns of conditioning.

A crucial feature or factor in this process is the presence of what Rogers termed 'the actualizing tendency', a tendency towards fuller and more complete personhood with an associated greater fulfilment of their potentialities. The role of the person-centred counsellor is to provide the facilitative climate within which this tendency can work constructively. 'The therapist trusts the actualizing tendency of the client and truly believes that the client who experiences the freedom of a fostering psychological climate will resolve his or her own problems' (Bozarth, 1998, p. 4). This is fundamental to the application of the person-centred approach. Rogers (1986, p. 198) wrote: 'the person-centred approach is built on a basic trust in the person . . . (It) depends on the actualizing tendency present in every living organism – the tendency to grow, to develop, to realize its full potential. This way of being trusts the constructive directional flow of the human being towards a more complex and complete development. It is this directional flow that we aim to release.'

The therapeutic relationship is central. A therapeutic approach such as person-centred affirms that it is not what you do so much as 'how you are' with your client that is therapeutically significant, and this 'how you are' has to be received by the client. Gaylin (2001, p. 103) highlights the importance of client perception. 'If clients believe that their therapist is working on their behalf – if they perceive caring and understanding – then therapy is likely to be successful. It is the condition of attachment and the perception of connection that have the power to release the faltered actualization of the self.' He goes on to stress how 'we all need to feel connected, prized – loved', describing human beings as 'a species born into mutual interdependence', and that there 'can be no self outside the context of others'. He highlights that 'loneliness is dehumanizing and isolation anathema to the human condition. The relationship', he suggests 'is what psychotherapy is all about.'

There is currently growing interest in, and much debate about, theoretical developments within the person-centred world and its application. Discussions on the theme of Rogers' therapeutic conditions presented by various key members of the person-centred community have recently been published (Wyatt, 2001; Haugh and Merry, 2001; Bozarth and Wilkins, 2001; Wyatt and Sanders, 2002). It seems to me that the relational component of the person-centred approach, based on the presence of the core conditions, is emerging strongly as a counter to the sense of isolation that frequently accompanies deep psychological and emotional problems, and the increase in what I would term a 'rabid inauthenticity' within materialistic societies as we enter the 21st century.

This is obviously a very brief introduction to the approach. Person-centred theory continues to develop as practitioners and theoreticians consider its application in various fields of therapeutic work and extend our theoretical understanding of developmental and therapeutic processes. At times it feels like it has become more than just individuals, rather it feels like a group of colleagues, based around the world, working together to penetrate deeper towards a more complete theory of the human condition. It is an exciting time.

CHAPTER 1

Background and review

It had been 11 months since Jennifer had begun attending the counselling sessions with Laura, her counsellor. She had felt depressed and had generally been feeling that life was just one big struggle. Over the next few months she had spent a lot of time looking at herself, how she behaved and why, and what she really wanted out of life.

Jennifer was 32 now and had had what she regarded as being a successful life in a great many ways. She had left school at 18 and had begun work for an advertising agency, initially as a secretary. She had stuck this for a couple of years before deciding to go to college on a part-time basis, undertaking a course in media and advertising. She had then worked for a variety of different agencies and had worked her way up to being an advertising consultant at one of the more prestigious companies.

In her personal life she had had relationships during that time, but had never really felt that she wanted to commit herself. Through her work she was involved in a lot of entertaining and it offered her a lot of social opportunities. The money was good, and she could afford to travel abroad regularly on exotic holidays.

It had therefore been something of a surprise to her in many ways when she had met Ian at an advertising promotional party. They had found themselves having so much in common – an interest in the theatre and the arts, an enjoyment of travel, an appreciation of good food. The list had seemed endless as they had chatted away over the buffet meal that evening. It hadn't been long before they had started living together. At first, they had commuted back and forth between their homes – they lived about 30 miles from each other. But later, Jennifer moved in with Ian and rented out her own home.

It had felt really good for a couple of years, but then she found that her mood had dipped. She had begun to lose interest in things and it was then that she approached Laura after finding her name in the British Association for Counselling and Psychotherapy Resources Directory. (This directory is updated annually and available from BACP – *see* Useful contacts.) She had also asked around and a friend had recommended Laura as well. This had left her feeling more reassured.

Laura offered counselling from her own home. She had her own dedicated counselling room and the house was detached so loud voices were not an issue.

The room was deliberately kept simple, but without having the feel of being devoid of stimulation. Bright pastel shades, a simple table and lamp, comfortable chairs and a couple of framed prints on the walls.

Working from home where there can be a problem with loud voices is an issue that does arise. Counsellors need to have thought this through and to be aware of it when they are working with clients who may feel unable to express themselves fully because of the feeling that they will disturb people. Where a person is clearly feeling unable to be themself because of this, then there is a need to discuss this and consider an alternative venue that will suit the client's needs.

Laura arranged to see Jennifer on Tuesday evenings, although this occasionally moved as circumstances demanded. Laura liked to offer a consistent time slot to her clients, but this was not always possible and both had agreed to work around this when necessary.

Jennifer had never done anything like this before, and it had felt strange at first. She had felt awkward, unsure of what to say, and sure that something wasn't quite right somehow. The way she kept describing it in the counselling sessions was 'something isn't right, but I can't get hold of what it is'. It frustrated her. Yet she had found over the months that Laura's listening and warm acceptance of her had somehow encouraged her to change. At least, her mood had lifted and she now had a much clearer sense of who she was. She had spent a lot of time looking at her lifestyle and how she had spent her time in recent years, and exploring what it was that felt unsatisfying.

One factor that had emerged in her counselling was her use of alcohol and cocaine. She had been a fairly heavy drinker for a number of years, really since her late teenage years. It had never become a problem to her, but she did tend to drink most days, up to a bottle of wine in an evening, sometimes more when at parties. A lot of this had gone with the job, but it continued when she was not at work or was on holiday. Alcohol had become a regular feature of her life, an important part of her relaxation at the end of a day, and her reward for the effort she put into her work.

The cocaine use had been more recent and had actually been a feature of a pressured advertising campaign. She had felt so energised by her cocaine use and had come to use it more and more. It had turned out that Ian had also used cocaine recreationally, although he seemed to have much less of a need for it. He seemed to be able to take it or leave it. But Jennifer had found herself needing to use it regularly.

Laura had been prepared to work with Jennifer on her cocaine and alcohol use. She didn't take on a role of a specialist drugs or alcohol counsellor, rather she treated it as another feature of Jennifer's lifestyle for her to bring to counselling if she wished to. She put no pressure on Jennifer to stop or cut back in any way, rather she allowed her to develop her own insight and understanding into her use, and to make her own decision to finally stop the cocaine and to cut back on the alcohol.

Jennifer had appreciated Laura's acceptance of her drug-using choices. It had felt like a huge thing to disclose, but she had begun to realise that the cocaine and alcohol use had become linked, giving her a rollercoaster of highs and lows which she had begun to find increasingly unmanageable. It had started out to be a great way of giving herself a boost to keep up with her work and it had really seemed to help the ideas flow to begin with, but eventually began to leave her struggling to come up with anything original.

She had stopped the cocaine, in fact she and Ian had decided together that they wanted it out of their lives. The mood swings that Jennifer experienced and the fact that it was a drain on their finances had led to them making this decision. At first, Jennifer's alcohol use had gone up but it had settled back down to a bottle a day. Now she had reduced further and she and Ian shared a bottle of wine each evening with their meal. Both felt comfortable with this, though there were times when Jennifer seemed to drink the bigger half of the bottle. And sometimes she might also have a gin afterwards, or a brandy, just to feel a warm glow into the latter part of the evening.

> Substance use and misuse is becoming an increasing feature of Western society and it is unrealistic for counsellors to expect to avoid clients using substances and/or seeking to resolve problems associated with past or present use. Basic drug and alcohol awareness can be helpful for the counsellor, not so that they can assume the role of expert within the counselling relationship, but simply to be informed and have some degree of confidence and credibility. It is also important that counsellors have approached this topic from a personal development angle, uncovering their own attitudes towards substance misuse in order to ensure that they have the capacity to offer unconditional acceptance, empathy and authenticity towards any client who may happen to be using substances, not necessarily as their primary problem, but more often as their way of coping with difficulties, pressures, stress and trauma.

Jennifer had been a regular attendee throughout the 11 months of counselling. So far they had had 32 sessions. The fact that the sessions would not always be weekly had been agreed in the initial counselling contract. Laura had felt comfortable with this. She could see that Jennifer was a busy woman and that she was fitting the counselling around other demands. Yet she was also mindful of not wanting to become simply 'a counsellor of convenience'. She recognised the importance and value of the therapeutic relationship that she formed with her clients, and recognised that consistent contact and a sense of commitment to the counselling process was important.

Laura had really grown to like Jennifer. She seemed to be quite a gutsy individual in many ways. Jennifer came across as being quite goal-orientated in her approach to life, and this certainly seemed to be reflected in her work, in which she was responsible for, or involved in, a succession of projects with clearly defined aims, objectives and target dates. However, as the counselling had continued she had noticed how Jennifer was becoming more laid back, more able to introduce other things into her life. One thing that Jennifer had gained from the counselling was a greater sense of spontaneity. Both she and Ian had found this a helpful change and it had freed them both up in many ways to make different and more satisfying choices in their lives.

Themes that Jennifer had been addressing recently in the counselling were issues concerning her relationship with her mother. She had rarely talked about her father, somehow he had always come across to Laura as being somewhat remote. But Jennifer certainly had issues with her mother and these largely revolved around her mother's tendency to keep interfering in Jennifer's life. She had been forever phoning up, asking questions about what Jennifer was doing, voicing her own opinions and generally leaving Jennifer with a sense that she couldn't please her mother whatever she did. The problem had eased. Jennifer had asserted her boundaries more and was less sensitive to her mother's comments. There were fewer tensions between them, although it was still not the easy-going relationship that Jennifer hoped for.

The difficulties had been around for a long time. As a child, Jennifer had always felt that her mother had been hypercritical of her, and had never really offered her the warmth she wanted. This had been a sharp contrast to Jennifer's younger sister, who always seemed to have received the love and attention that Jennifer had never really felt. She had talked a bit about her childhood, but more about the present and the challenges and struggles she was having in her adult life.

Angie, Jennifer's younger sister by two years, had taken quite a different direction in life. She had got married early to a chap she met whilst on holiday and had two children. Jack was now 7 and Susie was 4. They were great kids and Jennifer loved them both dearly. She saw them, but not as often as she would have liked. Angie now lived in Devon, a long way from Jennifer's home on the Sussex/Kent border. They would usually meet up at weekends five or six times a year, and for Christmas.

Jennifer kind of liked her sister, but it wasn't an easy relationship. Or at least that's how it had been for a long while. It had become easier more recently and Jennifer put this down to her counselling. She was finding herself less resentful of what Angie had received and she had not, in terms of her mother's affection.

Jennifer had come to realise that she could not change her mother, but that she could change her own reactions and behaviours. She recognised that the relationship had not been very good throughout her life, as far back as she could remember. She had distanced herself more from her mother, and contained the contact that they had. Jennifer had developed greater resilience to the criticism, realising that this negative conditioning had affected her and left her wanting to try to please her mother in a desperate attempt to receive the unconditional love that she now recognised she had been lacking and was still searching for. She realised that she was unlikely to gain what she wanted from her mother, and this had been incredibly painful for her, and it had taken many sessions to come to terms with this.

Much of our self-concept emerges from the interactions that we have with our parents and significant others in earlier life. The kind of negative conditioning that Jennifer has experienced is likely to have left her with a sense of self that might be summed up by the words 'I am unlovable' or 'no one hears my needs, I am invisible'. These beliefs, when re-enforced over time, become facts in the person's experience. Because they are aspects of the person's sense of self they then have to be satisfied in order to maintain psychological survival. So the person may then initiate actions and behaviours to re-enforce their negatively conditioned knowledge that they are unlovable, or invisible. Yet, at the same time, there will remain that part of them that yearns to be noticed and loved, creating an inner tension. The constant living out of the negatively conditioned sense of self creates a state of incongruence in the person, leaving them fundamentally anxious and to some degree fragmented.

So, it was now 11 months into the counselling and Jennifer did not have any sense of wanting to end it. She felt she was still gaining a great deal, learning about herself and discovering hidden traits that were the result of 'conditions of worth' from her past, and finding it valuable to have someone to talk to about issues that came up generally in her life – work, her relationship with Ian, general stresses and strains.

She had begun to feel more on top of things, somehow more in control of herself and her own direction in life. She was clearer about herself and what she wanted, and only recently she and Ian had been talking about starting a family.

Laura felt good about Jennifer's progress. She had gone through a tough time breaking her cocaine habit, but she had done it. She had stabilised her mood and had adjusted to her life with Ian, who seemed very supportive and caring. Laura had sensed shifts in her relationship with Jennifer as well. Laura was older than Jennifer, she was 48, and had ten years' experience in counselling. She had gained her diploma in person-centred counselling and psychotherapy and, whilst the course did address the issue of child sexual abuse, what really drew her interest was that during her training she had a placement at a rape and sexual abuse centre. This had involved further training additional to her diploma course. She later followed up with a module specifically focusing on working with survivors of abuse, not just sexual abuse. She did not feel that she was an expert on the topic, that had not been her purpose. Rather she regarded it as providing her with an opportunity to identify and work through her own issues and to gain an appreciation of the damage that arose and the impact sexual abuse could have on people both in childhood and later throughout their adult lives. It was not an issue that had arisen with Jennifer.

Looking back over the course of the counselling so far, Laura could see that something in Jennifer was settling down. The relationship had become less tense as time had gone on. This was not unusual, but at the beginning somehow there had seemed added tension with Jennifer and whilst Laura had highlighted this from time to time as she sought to achieve a congruent and transparent presence in the relationship, what it was had never really become clear. But it was easier now. The sessions still had a lot of emotional content, but not always. It felt comfortable but not to the point of being too cosy.

> With longer-term working, greater familiarity can develop, particularly where the counsellor is offering a relational therapy, one that sees the quality and nature of the therapeutic relationship as the primary factor that induces positive personality change. The division of counsellor–client can become less obvious and what can emerge is more of a genuinely person-to-person relationship. This can prove extremely valuable; however, the reality of counsellor–client remains and should not be lost sight of. Where counselling becomes overly conversational, or the sense of ease begins to obstruct congruent responses from the counsellor which, by their nature, are likely to be challenging or unsettling, then it needs addressing in supervision and in the sessions.

Laura was not sure how long Jennifer planned to stay in therapy. They had talked about it from time to time. On a recent occasion when this had come up, Laura had expressed her feelings about whether Jennifer might be experiencing some degree of dependence on her and, if so, what role this might have in Jennifer's life. 'No, I don't sense this as being dependence, but I do feel that I would miss it.' Further exploration revealed that what she thought she might miss most was the unconditional acceptance that she felt was present within the counselling space, and how that felt liberating for her to experience. 'It seems to help me to clarify for myself who I am without the interference of someone else's beliefs, agendas and angles. You seem to be very present but you do not kind of get in the way of me.'

It was now June, and Laura was aware that there would be breaks in the counselling. She took a break in August and she had already indicated this to Jennifer. Laura was also aware that Jennifer was planning to be away in late July.

> It is important for clients to be aware of this interruption to the flow of counselling. The person-centred counsellor will trust that the client, informed of a summer break, will adjust to this and take the necessary steps to prepare themselves. This could involve stepping back from in-depth work or avoiding particularly difficult or painful issues.

So, Jennifer has made a lot of progress over those 11 months and attends regularly. She has found ways of changing some of her habits and routines, she has learned to deal more effectively with her invasive mother and come to terms with the fact that her mother is unlikely to show her the affection that part of her has sought for so many years. She has a relationship with Ian that is going well and they are talking about starting a family. And Jennifer is less hassled by work and more able to give herself time to enjoy her life.

CHAPTER 2

Counselling session 33

It was 7.30pm and Laura was sitting in the counselling room waiting for Jennifer to arrive. The doorbell rang and it brought Laura back from her meditation on the colours in the sky as the sun reflected off the layers of cloud to the west. She smiled, got up and went down the hall to the front door to let Jennifer in.
'Hi,' Jennifer smiled, 'what a lovely evening. Feels nice and calm out there.'
'Yes, it is, I was just watching the colours in the sky myself. Come in.'

A bit of small talk is unavoidable in these circumstances, unless you wish to let the client in and maintain a silence, saying nothing until you enter into the therapy room. Perhaps some people follow this approach, but Laura wanted to communicate with her clients. She saw the conversation before entrance into the therapy room as part of the counselling process anyway. She was, after all, seeking to offer warm acceptance to Jennifer, to show she was attentive to what she was saying, and to offer her own presence as well. It established communication and contact, and for her this was a vital preliminary to the counselling session itself.

'So, how do you want to use our time this evening?' This was a common opening line that Laura used. She wasn't sure where she had picked it up from, but it had become her way of opening up the session when she had nothing particular that she wanted to say, or the client was not displaying signs of feelings that she could begin by empathically responding to.
Jennifer sat and thought for a moment or two. 'On my way over I was thinking about that, and then I got lost in looking out at the sky and the colours, and somehow everything seemed so peaceful. I didn't seem to see much traffic, not that there is much around here anyway. But it just all seemed, well, I don't know ... how can I put it?' She thought for a moment or two and Laura listened and waited attentively, not wanting to disturb Jennifer's process. 'It just felt good.'

'Mmmm,' Laura replied, and empathically reflected back, mirroring Jennifer's tone of voice, 'it just felt good.'

Jennifer smiled and was back with the image of the sky. The window in the counselling room looked south and from where she was sitting she couldn't see the same angle on the sun. 'Yes, I do feel good. It seems as though I have reached some kind of place of, I don't know . . . .' She stopped and thought again, trying to get a clear sense of what she was experiencing.

Laura sat and allowed Jennifer the time and space to do this. Over the period of time that they had been working together she had come to appreciate and respect Jennifer's style and way of being. She was a thinker and really liked to try to be precise about what she was feeling. She knew that Jennifer would be using the time so she sat attentively, waiting for her to respond with whatever insight emerged.

After about 30 seconds Laura noticed Jennifer suddenly nod her head and smile again. 'Yes, that's it. I feel as though I have reached some degree of self-acceptance. I guess I have been here before, but somehow it feels more substantial, more real, more me. I can't think of how else to put it.'

An emerging sense of self-acceptance is a vital element of an individual's process within the therapeutic context. Therapy is a path that takes the client through a series of key moments that bring an increasing sense of self-acceptance. These also seem to involve a sense of becoming at peace with oneself as issues are resolved and a fresh sense of self is integrated within the self structure. Often, however, each achievement is but a preparation for the emergence of some previously unseen aspect of oneself, some new element of incongruence that leaves the client unsettled.

Laura nodded. 'Mmmm. More self-accepting – more substantial, more real and more you.' Laura spoke slowly, allowing time for her empathic reflection to sink in as Jennifer listened. She had learned that this was a powerful way of communicating empathy.

Jennifer listened to Laura speaking, and yes, that was her. In particular the last two words stood out as Laura spoke them, 'more you'. Yes, she thought, that's it. 'More me, that really does sum it up. I kind of feel more whole, somehow, and I feel that my life is in a good place.'

Laura decided to reflect back Jennifer's actual words that she had used, 'more me, more whole and my life is in a good place'.

'Yes, and I really have to thank you for a lot of this. I mean, I really had some issues in my head when I started coming to see you, and, well, since then I feel I have really managed to get a grip on my life. And I'm kind of left wondering what to talk about now! I mean, counselling is supposed to be about talking through problems, but at the moment I don't really feel that I have any.'

'Mmmm.' Laura felt that Jennifer was flowing and didn't want to interrupt her with anything more than a minimal response.

'I've got a great weekend coming up. It's my niece's fifth birthday on Saturday and we are travelling down to Devon and having a long weekend at my sister's.'

Laura smiled and noted her curiosity about where exactly in Devon. She knew the area well, but knew that this would be a distraction. 'So, looking forward to the weekend?'

'Yes, and I'll be able to tell you about it next week. My niece's name is Susie. She's so sweet, so innocent. So much like me, how I was . . . .' Jennifer paused. She wasn't sure what was happening but she suddenly felt herself go cold. She shivered. She frowned, but didn't say anything.

Laura had noticed the frown and somehow the atmosphere had changed in the room. She felt concerned for Jennifer but she didn't know why. 'I noticed you frown.' And she added, 'Are you OK?' She hadn't meant to add the last bit but it just seemed to impel itself out of her mouth. She suddenly felt uneasy and realised that something was going on and that she needed to be very sensitive to herself and anything that Jennifer might want to communicate to her.

Jennifer heard Laura speak but she stayed sitting silently. She was still feeling cold but she did not know why. She didn't feel as though she had anything to say. She felt . . . how did she feel? She didn't exactly feel numb, and somehow she felt frozen but not icy. The silence continued. Jennifer just sat.

Laura felt she needed to respect Jennifer's silence. It had come about so suddenly. One minute Jennifer had been enthusing about her trip to Devon and seeing her niece, then a frown, and now silence. She thought about saying something to let Jennifer know that she was there, and that she didn't need to say anything unless she wanted to. Yet somehow that just felt like a line out of a textbook, contrived counsellor-speak. She wanted to trust that whatever was occurring for Jennifer in this moment was timely and necessary within herself.

An important feature of person-centred counselling is the recognition that the organismic self, the person, is essentially trustworthy when that person is offered the core conditions of unconditional positive regard, empathic responding and congruent expression. Here, Laura accepts that in some way Jennifer needs to be experiencing what is present for her. She does not know what it is, and at this point does not need to know. She offers her presence simply by being present with a focused attitude of warm attentiveness.

Jennifer knew Laura was there. She felt comforted knowing this, yet at the same time she knew she also felt distant. It seemed a contradiction, and she wasn't really thinking deeply about it, she just knew that Laura felt close and distant at the same time. But she wasn't thinking about Laura. The fact was that she wasn't thinking about anything. It seemed as though the world had stopped. Suddenly she felt herself taking a slow, deep breath, and as she did so she could feel the paralysis lifting. She blinked a few times and took a few more deep breaths. She was aware of having no sense of time, or of having experienced anything during that silence. Another deep breath and she looked at

Laura. 'I don't know what that was about. I have no idea how long I was in that silence.' Jennifer spoke the words quite softly.

Jennifer has entered into a dissociated state. Margaret Warner describes how young children, who experience severe early-childhood trauma and have not developed other ways of creating some distance from their experiences, can 'stumble on an ability to move into trance-like states that diminish immediate experiences of trauma'. She goes on to suggest that 'these trance-like states develop into clusters of experience that are subjectively experienced as independent selves' and that 'clients tend to move into such "parts" experiences when original trauma memories threaten to return. Such separate selves seem to offer a way to avoid being flooded by the original memories' (Warner, 2002).

Laura responded in a similar tone of voice as this felt like a sensitive moment. 'No idea . . . .' Laura let the words trail back into silence, allowing Jennifer the freedom to choose whatever she wanted to say about the experience.

'I went cold and I remember shivering, and then . . . I don't know. It was like I couldn't move, I couldn't think, I don't think I was feeling anything. I'm tempted to say it was like being a statue but that would be too heavy. I wasn't feeling heavy.' Jennifer paused.

Laura was about to respond when Jennifer began speaking again.

'No, I wasn't feeling heavy at all, but I wasn't feeling light either. I just wasn't feeling.' She spoke the words slowly and shook her head as she looked into Laura's eyes.

'You weren't feeling.' Laura kept her response simple, seeking to communicate back what she had heard and also offer the opportunity for Jennifer to stay with the experience should she wish to.

'No. I wasn't feeling anything. It was like my body was sitting here and I wasn't in it. No, that sounds ridiculous. I was in it, yet somehow, somehow . . . .' Jennifer shivered again. 'Ooh, that's weird.' She sat in silence for a moment.

'Weird?' Laura voiced her response as a question.

'It was . . . no, it's ridiculous, I mean.' Jennifer stopped again. 'You'll think I'm mad but, oh well, it's the only way I can describe it. It was as though my body was sitting here, I was looking out, but somehow I wasn't seeing anything. Yet I was, I mean I did see you, and the room, and everything, but there was a sense that I wasn't really *seeing* anything. Like nothing was coming back into my head.'

Laura nodded and responded empathically to Jennifer, seeking to accurately reflect what she was saying. 'As though your body was sitting there, you were looking out but not seeing anything.' She then ended with her last few words, 'Like nothing was coming back into your head.'

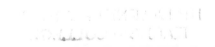

What is being described here could be taken literally or metaphorically. It is not fully understood by the client and she is struggling to convey in words what she has experienced. Where this is the case, it is important for the counsellor to convey accurately their empathic understanding of what is being said. It can be a sensitive time and the client could be easily impressed by some other perspective that a less empathically sensitive counsellor might offer, or a more open or loose empathic response that leaves the client feeling unheard, both of which could have the effect of diminishing the client's own tenuous attempt to describe and make sense of their experience. Warner (2000) emphasises how she would use the client's same words when empathically responding to a client who is describing something that could be metaphorical and connected to some dissociative process, and which often sounds odd or disconnected in some way.

Jennifer nodded slowly. She felt very different somehow but she did not know how to describe it. Like feeling and non-feeling at the same time. It didn't make sense. But this was what was happening inside her, to her.

'I feel so close to that experience, Laura, so close. It's like it's inside me, part of me . . . .' Again Jennifer's voice tailed off as she shook her head slightly from side to side and took another deep breath. 'Is this making any sense?'

Perhaps Laura could make sense of it, but this would probably only lead into some kind of intellectual exchange over what might be the theoretical cause of what Jennifer had been, and to some degree still was, experiencing. What Laura was more interested in was in helping Jennifer to understand for herself what she was experiencing. It was her experience and for someone else to interpret it or try to make sense of it could miss the point. And besides, her role as a person-centred counsellor was not to make sense of her client's experiences for them, but rather to stay in a therapeutic relationship with them as they explored their inner world.

Laura responded to what Jennifer had said about her experience and acknowledged her wish to know whether what she was saying was making sense. 'It's so close, inside you, a part of you.'

'Yes, part of me.' Jennifer lapsed back into silence. A sentence had formed inside her head and it made her feel uncomfortable.

Laura noticed Jennifer frown again, but she was also struck by what Jennifer had chosen to acknowledge in response to what she, Laura, had just said. 'Part of you. And I notice that whatever you are experiencing is making you frown,' she responded, empathising with Jennifer's facial expression.

Jennifer nodded, breathed deeply and sighed. 'A phrase came into my head just as I was speaking and it left me feeling uncomfortable.'

'Mmmm, uncomfortable,' Laura nodded gently and waited. She wanted to leave Jennifer to decide whether she was prepared to share this sentence.

Jennifer sat pondering on the phrase. Somehow she didn't want to hear herself say it. It was uncomfortable enough to think it, but to say it. It felt .... She was suddenly aware of her heart beating, well actually it was thumping and she could feel herself beginning to sweat a little. Suddenly she felt very warm, and her heart continued to thump. She breathed deeply and tried to open her mouth. But her lips wouldn't move. The heartbeat seemed to have increased and she could sense a kind of roaring in her ears. She suddenly felt very faint.

Laura felt something happening in the atmosphere. It suddenly felt quite electric. She had noticed that Jennifer had momentarily looked as if she wanted to say something, and that her breathing had suddenly seemed to go quite deep and fast. Now she .... Oh no, she thought, what's happening?

Jennifer had slumped back into the chair and her eyes had closed.

'Jennifer? Are you OK? Can you hear me? Jennifer?' Oh God, Laura thought, she's passed out. She reached over and took Jennifer's hand, patting her gently but firmly on the wrist. 'Jennifer, are you OK? Jennifer? Can you hear me?'

Jennifer suddenly took a deep breath and opened her eyes. 'What happened? It's hot in here.'

'You fainted. Let me open the window and let in some fresh air.' Laura stood up and went over to the window, opening it outwards and immediately feeling a rush of cool air. She returned to her seat.

'Oh, that feels good.' Jennifer took in a few deep breaths and reached over to the glass of water that was on her side of the coffee table. She took a mouthful and swallowed it slowly, then another, and returned the glass to the table. 'I remember being aware that my heart was thumping and I tried to say something but my lips wouldn't move. The next thing I knew you were holding my hand and calling my name.'

'Well, it's OK now. Just take your time. No need to rush anything. How are you feeling?' Laura was deliberately stepping out of counselling mode. She wanted to be sure that Jennifer was OK. 'Do you have fainting attacks?'

'No, I don't recall anything like that. I just remember my heart thumping away and a kind of roaring sound in my ears. Then nothing. Was I out for long?'

'Seconds.'

'Sorry.' Jennifer was very aware of the look of concern on Laura's face. She felt she must have really worried her.

'That's OK.' Laura smiled.

Jennifer suddenly yawned. 'My goodness, I suddenly feel really tired.' She yawned again, and then reached out for the glass of water, drinking most of what was left before returning it to the table.

Laura was wondering whether the fainting attack had been connected to what Jennifer had been experiencing or had appeared to have been trying to say. Yet she also didn't want to bring the focus back to therapy straight away as she felt Jennifer needed to regain her own focus.

'No need to say anything Jennifer, just take your time. Can I top up your water for you?'

'Yes please.'

Laura picked up the glass and went out to the kitchen. When she returned she found that Jennifer had got up and was stretching with her hands above her head. 'I had to get up and stretch. I was suddenly aware of feeling tight across my back and in my shoulders. My legs felt a bit wobbly but I've got my balance again now.' She yawned again as she tried another stretch. 'Oh dear, sorry about that.' She smiled, twisted her back to the right and the left and then returned to her seat.

'Do you want to continue with the session, Jennifer? I guess I am saying that because I am unsure how you are feeling and what you feel your needs are at this moment.'

'I don't really feel that I can focus on much just at the moment. I feel like I want to head back home and have an early night. I just feel so tired, absolutely drained. Do you mind?'

Laura has taken the decision to raise the issue as to whether Jennifer wants to complete the whole session. She trusts that Jennifer knows what her needs are and wants her to have the opportunity to respond to what is present for her. She also wants to convey her concern and caring.

'No, not at all.' Laura was aware of a concern she was feeling and thought that it was appropriate and responsible to voice it. 'Do you think you should see someone, your GP for instance, about having fainted like that?'

'I'll see how I feel in the morning. I think that I just got a bit intense somehow and ....' Her voice tailed off, but she continued, 'I'll be OK. I had a busy day today. I didn't have a chance to eat before coming over either, maybe that had something to do with it. I'll take it easy driving back. I don't have far to go and I am feeling a bit clearer now, but I will just sit for a moment or two longer.'

'OK. Look, I would appreciate it if you could give me a call when you get back home to let me know you got back safely? I'm just concerned in case you have another fainting attack.'

'I'll be OK. I'm feeling a lot better already. I think I've overdone it today and it's caught up with me.' As she finished her sentence she felt a yawn coming on and could do nothing to stifle it. 'Sorry.'

'Seems like that tiredness is going to grab your attention one way or another.'

'Yes. But that stretch just now was good, got me back into my body.' Jennifer frowned for a moment. 'That was a funny thing to say. But that was what it felt like. Anyway, can I just take a minute or two more to finish this water and then I'll head off.'

Laura thought about picking up on her comment, but was mindful that Jennifer had made it clear that she was heading off and she wanted to respect that. 'Sure, take whatever time you need.' Laura wanted to acknowledge what had been said but without entering back into counselling mode. So she added, 'Seems like this experience has given you something to think about.'

'Yes, strange that. Back into my body. Oh well.' Jennifer stood up. She felt a lot steadier now. 'Same time next week?'

'Yes, sure.' Laura was still feeling concerned, but the colour had returned to Jennifer's cheeks.

'Great. And I'll tell you about the weekend. And I'll also let you know if I make any sense of what happened earlier in the session.' Jennifer paused momentarily. 'Strange.' She shook her head, sat back down again and reached into her handbag to take out her chequebook. She wrote her cheque out to Laura for the session and handed it to her.

'Thanks, are you sure you are OK?' She had noticed that Jennifer had stood up, forgetting momentarily about the cheque, and was wondering how focused she was for driving back home.

'Yes, but I appreciate your concern.' Jennifer stood up, as did Laura, who followed her out of the room.

'So, see you next week. Thanks for that session, I'm not yet sure what it was all about but I do feel I need an early night. Maybe we can take another look at it next week, and I'll promise not to faint next time!'

Laura smiled, although she knew she still felt concern. Something was going on and she needed to talk it through with her supervisor before she next saw Jennifer. Fortunately her next supervision session was at the end of the week. Laura opened the door for Jennifer to leave. 'Thanks again, and see you next week. Bye.'

'Bye Jennifer. Take care.'

'Will do.'

Laura stood for a moment and watched Jennifer heading for her car. She was walking steadily and confidently. Maybe she was worried about nothing. But there was something distinctly odd about that session. She sensed that more had been going on than had been talked about. The transition from talking about the trip to her sister's and her niece's birthday and that silence, and her sense that Jennifer had been trying to say something just before she fainted. Dammit, she suddenly thought, and I still don't know what she had been trying to say. Oh well, if it is important I'm sure it will come back again. Trust the process . . . .

Supervision

Laura met up with Malcolm for supervision of her client work every month. She did not talk about all of her clients at each session, but chose those who felt most pressing, or caused her to feel unsure about something. She did, however, ensure that over a period of two supervision sessions she had mentioned her work with all of her clients at least once.

How a counsellor decides which clients to bring to supervision is an issue. To only go with those who seem pressing can mean that some never get mentioned, and this is not good practice. Sometimes the client about whom a counsellor feels they have no issue to bring to supervision is the one with whom they have become too comfortable and perhaps are missing important features of the counselling interaction. Supervision is not only about addressing problems or difficulties. It can also offer the opportunity to simply explore the content of sessions or the counsellor's experience of working with a client to deepen their appreciation and understanding of what is occurring. Supervision can also be a place in which to acknowledge and celebrate a client's growth and development and the role that the counsellor has played in that process.

Laura wanted to spend time discussing Jennifer. She could still recall quite vividly the image of Jennifer slumped in the chair, the colour drained from her face. And she had this sense of something having been unsaid. Anyway, she had decided to begin by talking about Jennifer.

'I want to say something about my last session with Jennifer. It was ....' Laura thought for a moment. 'It was certainly interesting.' She hadn't really been able to find the word she wanted.

'Interesting?' Malcolm replied, with a slight tilting of his head and the raising of his eyebrows.

'Yes,' Laura smiled, 'I know you know that I often say that word when I'm at a loss for what to say. But it was interesting and I really do need to try to make sense of it. I feel as though I am missing something or, at least, something is being kept hidden from me. I have been thinking about it since the session and somehow I just sense something is happening, but I'm wondering whether Jennifer is aware yet of what it is. Am I making much sense here?' Laura felt that she had been rambling a bit.

'What I hear you saying is that you need to make sense of that last session, that you were left with a sense that something was hidden and you are now unsure whether or not Jennifer is aware of what that something is. Does that sound right, and does that make sense to you?'

'Yes, it does. I guess the bit that leaves me feeling uncertain or confused is this nagging sense that there is something else happening but I don't know what it is.' Laura was aware that she wasn't telling Malcolm what happened, but was getting more tangled up in what she did not know rather than what she did.

'Mmmm, something else going on but you can't get hold of what it is.' Malcolm spoke the words slowly to give Laura time to reflect on them. He could see the concentration on her face. She looked as though she was struggling to get hold of something but it just wasn't making itself clear to her. He voiced what he was experiencing. 'You look as though you are really concentrating and trying to get hold of this something, but it just won't make itself visible to you.'

'Can't get hold of it. So let's just accept that there is a something and maybe if I talk more about what happened I'll be able to come back to it and get another angle on it.'

Acknowledging the presence of a 'something' can sometimes be all that can be achieved. It is as though there is some kind of presence on the edge of awareness, a bit like having a sense that there is something just over the horizon yet it is not yet visible. A little more of the journey is required before it can begin to appear and enter into awareness.

Malcolm nodded.

'So, the last session. Jennifer came feeling very positive and seemed to be struggling to know what to say. She began talking about her niece whose birthday is coming up this weekend, and how she is going down to Devon for it. She seemed very enthusiastic and it all felt really good.' Laura frowned as she thought back to what had happened next. 'Then it was strange. She began talking about her niece and was saying something about how she was just like her when she was . . . and she didn't finish the sentence, but went very quiet, and I mean, very quiet. The atmosphere changed. I asked if she was OK but she didn't respond. Eventually she came out of it, after a few minutes had passed.'

Malcolm was aware that the atmosphere had changed in the room as Laura had been speaking. It had become more intense. He commented on it. 'I am aware that this feels more intense all of a sudden.'

'Yes, and it was intense at the time.' Laura sunk her chin into her right hand and reflected back on the experience. 'Jennifer just sat. She said afterwards that it had felt weird, as though she was looking out through her eyes but taking nothing in. She said she couldn't remember feeling anything and yet feelings were present. And she added that she felt the experience remained close to her, that she felt she could easily slip back into it.'

'How did it feel for you to be with her in that experience?'

'It didn't feel like a normal working silence, or the kind of awkward silence that occurs when a client doesn't know what to say next. It was neither of those.' Laura stopped again and thought for a moment. Malcolm allowed her the space to continue with her train of thought, deciding not to disturb the flow of experiencing that was present for Laura. He simply nodded and waited.

'She described it as feeling like being a statue, but then she said that it wasn't like a heavy kind of statue, yet she also said she hadn't felt light either. There just seemed to be so many paradoxes in what she was experiencing. As I think back now I can see her sitting there and it was as though she wasn't really there. I mean, she was, but somehow it felt as though she wasn't. It was very powerful. It left me feeling a little light-headed. It seemed incredibly important somehow even though I am still not sure what it was all about.'

Malcolm nodded again. 'So, it left you feeling light-headed and seemed incredibly important. Was it hard to stay with her then?'

'No, it wasn't hard, it just felt strange somehow.' Laura's thoughts went back to what Jennifer had been saying before it had all happened. 'I'm thinking back to what had led up to it. She had been talking about her niece, Susie, as I mentioned. Something about being like her, and I think she was going to say that she was like her when she was Susie's age. And then off she went inside herself.' Laura could feel herself stiffen. 'Something happened, Malcolm, something happened to Jennifer and I don't know what it is, but her thinking of Susie took her to somewhere in herself, a place where she stopped thinking, feeling and seeing.' Laura felt goose bumps breaking out over her arms and neck. 'Yes, I hadn't put that together before now. She stopped thinking, feeling and seeing. She said she was looking out but nothing was coming back in.' Laura frowned. 'Makes me want to shiver,' and as she said this she felt a shiver run through her body.

'It really affects you, Laura, it's got into your body. How does it feel?' Malcolm recognised that bodily experiences could often reflect psychological content and could often shed light on what was happening within a therapeutic situation.

'It doesn't feel good. Feels like I want to shake something off. Yes, that's how I felt when I shivered. I wanted to shake something off.'

'Shake something off,' Malcolm reflected back, aware that he had emphasised the word 'something'.

'Back to the "something".' Laura sought to be open to what was present for her in her feelings and in her body. 'There's still nothing I can get hold of. Just a sense but no clear definition to what it is I'm sensing. I don't think I'm going to get hold of it, not yet anyway.'

'You think it may simply be out of reach?'

'Yes. But this isn't the end of the story.' The image of Jennifer sitting there having passed out had come vividly back into her thoughts. 'There was something that Jennifer was trying to say. She had come out of that silent, not thinking-feeling-seeing state, and she said something about some phrase that had come to mind, but she never said what it was, and I didn't ask her. What happened next was that Jennifer suddenly fainted in the chair.'

Malcolm was aware of concern present inside himself, both for Jennifer who had clearly gone through an incredibly intense experience if it had triggered some kind of fainting fit, and for Laura who had had to deal with the situation at a time when she would have been straining to keep her senses open and receptive to whatever Jennifer sought to communicate to her. He felt a temptation to ask her how she had handled it, but realised quickly that this would take Laura away from processing her thoughts and feelings, her internal reactions to what had happened. He noted the temptation and stepped aside from it.

Directing a supervisee towards practical considerations could sometimes be a defence by the supervisor to avoid engaging with something difficult. These can be returned to. The initial emphasis should be on the supervisee's processing of their experience. For the person-centred supervisor much emphasis will be placed on how the supervisee's congruence and positive regard is affected by working with a client, with particular emphasis on what effect that might be having on the supervisee's ability to be sensitively and accurately empathic. Supervision, from a person-centred way of work-ing, is going to be focused more on the supervisee than on the client. The aim is to help to ensure that the supervisee is able to enter into a therapeutic relationship with the client with the minimum of distortion or blockage to their accurate experiencing and expression of what is being communicated to them.

'That must have triggered off a lot of feelings and thoughts for you?' Malcolm
   sought to hold the focus on Laura's internal experiencing.
'Anxiety. In that moment when I realised what had happened I felt an adrenalin
   rush and my heart began thumping. It had never happened to me before.
   I called her name and asked if she could hear me, but I got no response.
   I instinctively reached out to her hand, held her wrist and tapped gently but
   firmly. I kept talking to her and she came out of it. It was totally instinctive. Thank God she did come round.' She took a deep breath. 'Doesn't bear
   thinking about.'
'Anxiety, leaving you with a vivid memory and a real sense of gratitude that
   she came round.' Malcolm was feeling very warm towards Laura as he spoke
   these words. He appreciated what a shock it must have been and voiced this.
   'Quite a shock.'
'It was. It really was. And it only lasted a few seconds but it seemed to last for an
   age. Time seemed to just get stretched. When she came round she said she had
   felt her heart thumping and a roaring in her ears and then she was aware of
   my voice.'
'And you said something about her having been trying to speak before it happened?'
'Yes, and I thought about asking her but she was very drained and somehow it
   didn't feel quite right to me to go back into therapeutic mode. I pulled back.
   I guess I was concerned and didn't want to put her under any strain, and I
   wanted to let her decide if she wanted to tell me something. But she never did.
   So I'm still at a loss to know what she had been thinking and had been wanting to say. I'm sure it's all connected. Right from mentioning her niece and
   going into that conscious non-thinking-feeling-seeing state, and then passing
   out completely.'
Laura shook her head and as she did so a thought struck her quite forcibly.
   'I think she was going to say something important.' She could feel the goose
   bumps again. 'I think that when she reacted to talking about her niece she
   entered into some deep part of herself, and I think it is a traumatised place
   struggling to find its voice.' The goose bumps had now spread down her back

and into her neck. 'I think she passed out because some part of her was about to find its voice and the only way for other parts of her to stop it was to shut her down. I think there is a five-year-old girl inside Jennifer who wants to tell us something, but other parts of her are frantically trying to stop her from speaking.' Laura was looking into Malcolm's eyes and she could feel tears welling up in her own. 'Something terrible happened, Malcolm.' The goose bumps had spread to her legs now. 'Something terrible happened.'

This notion that a person can have within them many voices, often in conflict, and perhaps working together to maintain a secret, can be a feature of traumatic experience. Warner (2000, pp. 160–61) writes of how 'children almost always divide the dissociated aspects of their experiences into a number of compartments that are separate from each other'. She later adds that a number of these dissociated parts can take on self-abusive or suicidal qualities, 'impulses that arise when the pain of dissociated memories threatens to return'. The fainting attack could be regarded as a means whereby Jennifer's body sought to block out the emergence of a memory that was getting close to breaking into her everyday awareness.

Malcolm also felt the intensity of the moment and the unease that seemed to have become very present as Laura had been speaking. 'You look very tearful, Laura, it's really affecting you.' He responded to what Laura was feeling rather than the content of what she had been talking about.

Laura had taken out a tissue and was brushing away tears. 'She has never alluded to anything. But there was something different about that session as though something was trying to surface and it got close. I think that her visit to Devon is going to be quite significant and I am really aware of not knowing what to expect from our next session.'

Malcolm was wondering what Laura was feeling might be the nature of the experience seeking to emerge within Jennifer's awareness. 'What do you sense might happen?'

'I think that whatever is happening for Jennifer may get intensified, maybe other memories may surface and perhaps she will become quite distressed. It seems she is dissociating as a defence against this emergence. I sense a really difficult time coming up for her and just as we are heading into summer when we both know that there will be gaps in the counselling because of our respective holidays.'

'Do you trust Jennifer to be able to hold things together?'

'I don't know. In a way, yes, I do believe that unresolved traumas surface when the time is right, when psychologically they can no longer be held back and often at a time when the person can deal with them, albeit it is a very painful process often requiring lots of appropriate support.' Laura stopped for a moment.

Malcolm was thinking about Laura and her needs, whether she felt she was getting enough support to face what seemed likely to be a very distressing phase in
her therapeutic relationship with Jennifer. 'What about you? What are or will
be your needs?'

'I think I might be bringing Jennifer to supervision more regularly, in fact, I am
sure that I will be.' Laura thought for a moment. 'I'm glad that Jennifer and I
have been working together for almost a year. I think the relationship is
strong and perhaps that is contributing to this part of Jennifer feeling able or
ready to be heard. It feels good to have talked about all of this. I don't want to
carry preconceived ideas into the session, I want to keep my mind and feelings
open so that I can genuinely hear what Jennifer has to say and to experience
whatever is present without having some expectation to contrast it with.
I don't want to analyse it further at this time. I feel more comfortable with my
anticipation that at some point in the next few weeks some new material will be
brought into the counselling, and that I need to be very focused and warmly
accepting of whatever it is that Jennifer discloses. Whatever she says won't be
easy, but I feel more ready to hear it. Somehow talking about this ''something''
has made it feel ... , I don't know, I feel able to accept it because we have
acknowledged its presence even if we haven't defined it.'

Malcolm nodded. 'Feel you are in a different place with it, more accepting and the
thought that comes to my mind is that maybe there is a greater sense of connection, the ''something'' is no longer right on the edge of awareness. It is
unclear but it is somehow more present even though we can only refer to it as
a ''something''.'

'Yes. Yes, I feel calmer. Anxious about how it will be for Jennifer, and for me, but
somehow calmer as well. Thanks for that. I feel I need to move on now to two of
my other clients. But I know we'll be talking about Jennifer again next time.'

The supervision session moved on. At the end of the session Malcolm was aware
that he was still left with his own speculations concerning Jennifer. He knew
that he, like Laura, must be focused and present.

Through the process of talking about her client and her experience of what
occurred in the session, Laura has been able to connect, during this supervision session, with her own sense of anxiety and the sense that something
is emerging within Jennifer. She voices her concern as to whether Jennifer
can 'hold it together'. The fact that what has occurred could be the first indicator of a dissociative process within Jennifer, with the very real possibility
that aspects within that dissociative process could be self-abusing or self-
harming, should rightly trigger concern for the client's wellbeing. However,
for the person-centred counsellor the challenge is not to let that concern
obstruct their ability to maintain empathic contact with the client, to offer
warm acceptance of all dissociate parts that may emerge (even the destructive ones) and to trust that the client's process of actualisation will take her
towards a more satisfying, fulfilling and congruent way of being.

Points for discussion

- What do you think is happening within Jennifer, and how would you explain this in terms of person-centred theory?
- What feelings and thoughts become present for you when contemplating the possibility of a client passing out during a counselling session?
- Should Laura have pressed Jennifer to voice whatever it was that she had thought prior to fainting?
- Was it appropriate to end the session early? What would be the relative pros and cons of staying with the therapeutic process?
- What were the key moments within the counselling session with Jennifer?
- In supervision, speculation as to the nature of the 'something' that has become present in Jennifer's edge of awareness did not lead to anything definite. Was this appropriate use of supervision, or should it have moved towards trying to name the 'something'?
- Where do you feel the balance should lie in supervision between focusing on what is happening for the client and what has become present for the supervisor?
- Did Laura receive from the supervision the kind of responses that you would have wanted had you been her?
- Evaluate both the counselling and supervision sessions from a person-centred perspective.

CHAPTER 3

Counselling session 34

'I want to ask how you were after last session, but I also want to leave you free to use this time to focus on whatever you wish to focus on.' Laura wanted to express her genuine concern as she was still very aware of how intense that last session had been.

'A bit wobbly at first. I still don't really understand it all. I had a bad night after the last session, I couldn't settle. I don't know what that was about. One of those really restless nights. Ian said I was all over the bed. I felt troubled somehow but I didn't know what about. I remember waking up at one time feeling really uneasy, really anxious, mega-butterflies in my stomach and my heart pounding. But I don't remember dreaming anything, and I didn't have any thoughts in my mind when I woke up. The next day at work was a struggle. I actually came away early and had a sleep when I got home. That's not like me, but I had to.'

'So, this kind of disturbed sleep and then feeling tired and needing to sleep the next day was quite out of character.'

'Very much so. It sort of happened again a little bit the next night, but not so intense, and then we drove down to Devon for the long weekend. I seemed to sleep OK down there, although the first night I was unsettled, but then I usually am on the first night when I go away.'

'So, one more slightly disturbed night, then Devon.' Laura decided to be brief, not sure whether Jennifer would wish to stay with the disturbed sleep or describe her trip.

'Yes. I had a great time. Susie and her brother really enjoyed themselves, and so did I. We drove down on the Friday and were there mid-afternoon. We relaxed a bit, went out with the children to a nearby beach for a couple of hours. Had ice cream and generally messed around. Ian took them crabbing in the rock pools. They got a couple of weeny ones and got very wet in the process! But they enjoyed it. I had a nice chat with my sister, and that seemed to go really well.' Jennifer was smiling and was feeling quite comfortable talking about it. She could still feel the relaxed nature of the weekend. She felt good.

'Sounds like a really good time and a bit of a holiday for everyone.'

'Yes, it was, and I realised how much I needed it. I was more tired than I thought I was. I had the energy to be involved, but by the evenings each day I was aware that I was flagging. Had a few more drinks than I probably should have each evening, but I was OK. No, it felt good and I am pleased to have gone down to see them. Susie really loved the presents we had taken, and that was great too.'

Laura noticed the urge to ask what presents Susie had been given but let it go. Her curiosity, not a therapeutic need. 'Tiring but good, and a little too much to drink.'

'Sums it all up pretty well.'

Jennifer spent a large part of the rest of the session talking more about what they had done over the weekend and about some of the conversations she had had with her sister. It had all felt very comfortable and they had agreed that they would plan a holiday together sometime the following year. Towards the end of the session Jennifer made a reference to the previous session. 'I'm feeling more like the me that I was before that last counselling session. I don't know what that was about, whether I had an off day, was a bit over-stressed or over-tired. I certainly must have been more tired than I thought given how I felt at times when I was away. Yet I do still go over parts of that session in my mind. It doesn't disturb me, I think I can make sense of it. I think I was just tired, it was a hot day and I lost my concentration.' Jennifer had reflected on it and genuinely felt this way about it.

Laura heard what Jennifer was saying and was aware that she could be tempted to introduce her concerns, but it was clear that this was not appropriate.

The person-centred counsellor trusts her client's process and believes that if something is to be acknowledged then it would arise in its own good time. The counsellor's role is to provide the therapeutic conditions as Rogers had suggested: congruence, empathy and unconditional positive regard, and allow the client's own actualising tendency to promote within her the growth towards fuller awareness of her structure of self.

'Sounds as though you have made sense of it for yourself, a hot day and you were tired. So it isn't disturbing you, although you find that you still think about it?'

'I do think about it. I guess what puzzles me is the sense of not knowing. I mean, when I went into that silent state of non-thinking and non-feeling, well, it was so weird. And then passing out like that. I remember a sense of feeling paralysed, but I can't remember when that happened, and trying to explain how I felt.'

Laura felt a moment of recognition. Yes, that's what Jennifer had been trying to say before she passed out, something about feeling paralysed. 'I think it was before you passed out. You had looked as though you were trying to say something. I think it was then.'

'Ooh, makes me shiver again thinking about it. Talking to you about it makes it feel more real. Or maybe it is being in this room.' Jennifer felt a wave of unease again, deep in her stomach. It was fleeting and was fading again. She didn't say anything. She didn't feel that she wanted to get back into it. 'Anyway, I feel OK now.' In fact she knew she didn't but she really felt she wanted to get back to the good feelings she had been experiencing earlier when recounting the story of her weekend.

> Jennifer is in a state of incongruence. What she is communicating is not reflecting her experience. Anxiety will be present. It feels too uncomfortable for her to contemplate engaging with her unease and she is denying it to Laura although within herself she knows it is present.

Laura was aware that part of her was back in her supervision session and was wondering what may have happened to Jennifer in the past, whilst another part was listening to her saying she was feeling OK. She was aware of the gulf between the two parts of herself. It persisted. 'You feel OK, really OK?' Laura said this with the added emphasis on *really* to reflect what Jennifer was saying but also to provide Jennifer with the opportunity of engaging with what she was feeling. If Jennifer continued to say she was OK whilst consciously denying to Laura that she was not feeling OK, then this would probably increase her discomfort and anxiety due to her incongruent state. However, in reflecting back what Jennifer had said, Laura was also offering her the opportunity, if she genuinely was feeling OK, to affirm this. Either way, the client can connect with her feelings whilst reserving the right to communicate what she wishes the counsellor to hear.

'Yes, I'm OK.' As she said it, she could feel her heart thumping again. She knew that something was not OK, but she didn't want to go back into that weird experience as in the previous session. She sought to look composed as she spoke.

'OK.' Laura let it go. Jennifer clearly wanted her to hear that she was OK, and so she decided to acknowledge that. She also knew what she was feeling inside, but decided not to voice it.

> There is a common misconception that congruence means that the counsellor says anything and everything that she may be feeling or thinking. When a client is working with incongruence, however, and for reasons of discomfort is choosing not to communicate something to the counsellor, then it can simply lead to a whole succession of challenges by the counsellor on what the client is saying. This is not a person-centred way of working. What the client communicates is accepted and respected. She is telling the counsellor what she wants heard. The person-centred counsellor will express what she is experiencing where it is pressing or obstructing their ability to listen to the client, and this experience is emerging out of empathic sensitivity to what the client is seeking to convey.

In this example, Laura has accepted that at this point Jennifer wants her to hear that she is OK. She respects this. Nevertheless, she is aware of feeling a split in herself and will bear this in mind as possibly being linked to a possible split in the client. Where there is a definite gulf between what the client is saying and what the client is experiencing, the counsellor can find themselves split as well, one aspect of themselves attending to the words being spoken, another to what is being sensed that is unspoken. The importance of accurate self-awareness and congruence in the counsellor enables them to recognise experiences that are likely to have relevance to the therapeutic relationship and what is present for the client.

Jennifer looked up at the clock, the session was nearly over. She felt some relief inside her. 'I feel like this is a good place to end the session. You know that I can't make it next week – work commitments, we discussed it a couple of weeks back. I forgot to mention it last time with everything that happened.'

'Yes. So I shall see you again in two weeks.'

'Yes. I'm not sure what I will use the session to focus on. Maybe I don't need to keep coming so often now?'

Laura sensed that Jennifer was perhaps trying to end the sessions. This felt all rather abrupt somehow and, on the back of what she had been saying about being OK, it didn't feel comfortable. She decided to let Jennifer know that she had heard what she had said. 'So, you are wondering whether to come as often. Maybe that is something we could talk about next time as it is so close to the end of this session. Maybe we can review things a bit at the next session?'

'That sounds good. And we can decide what my options are. Yes.' Jennifer could feel her heart thumping again. It did not feel at all comfortable. She took the cheque out of her handbag as she was speaking. 'See you in two weeks at the same time.'

'Thanks. Yes.' The session ended and Laura walked to the door with Jennifer and let her out. When she had gone she went back into the counselling room and just sat for a while. Something was going on, she said to herself. Something is trying to be heard and something else is trying to stop it, and it is ready to urge Jennifer to stop coming to achieve this. After a few minutes Laura got up and went to her desk to write up her notes. 'Something', the word was very present for her. 'Something', she heard herself say out loud, 'something, but what is it?'

It seems highly likely that part of Jennifer is seeking to sabotage the counselling in order to avoid what is currently hidden to her experience from surfacing. It is as though a part of her is seeking to silence another part which is coming close to finding its voice. Laura was right to feel uneasy about what she was experiencing as a potentially rather abrupt ending. Something was indeed going on.

Counselling session 35

It was a fortnight later and Jennifer had arrived on time for her counselling session feeling disturbed. She did not understand what was happening to her, or why, but she knew that she was feeling distinctly uncomfortable and anxious. She was glad of the hour with Laura to begin to try to make sense of things.

'So,' Laura began, 'I know we talked of using some of the time today as a kind of review, but I also want to be open to anything else more pressing that you might wish to talk about.'

Jennifer was feeling quiet, almost withdrawn in herself. It felt as though her intention to talk of her discomfort was being, well, kind of pushed away. She wanted to talk about it but somehow the urgency seemed to have receded. Yet she also knew it was there. She heard herself say, 'Yes, a review, good idea.' She paused and looked up. 'What do you think?'

Laura was aware of feeling strangely out of touch with Jennifer, it felt as though Jennifer was not fully present for her, and this was not her usual experience. Jennifer seemed distant to Laura, or rather perhaps she should more rightly own her sense of being distant from Jennifer. It felt very strong and she sensed it was important to voice her experience as well as convey her empathy for what Jennifer had just said.

Laura decides to be not only empathic to what Jennifer has said, but also to the sensed presence of something else. Laura's awareness of herself and how she experiences being with Jennifer has meant that something different has stood out in sharper relief and Laura does not feel it is coming from her. She voices it.

'You think a review is a good idea, and I am also aware of experiencing you as quite distant somehow. Not sure what it's about, but I just wanted to let you know.'

Jennifer stayed silent and did not respond. To Laura, she seemed very small, yet she wasn't really. She noted the experience and sensed that something must be happening and that she should allow it to continue and to become present at its own pace, whatever *it* was. The silence continued. Laura was aware of a growing discomfort within herself and she knew herself well enough to know that this was not her usual experience of being in silence with a client. Quite a few minutes had passed and Jennifer had continued looking down, making no movement and no eye contact. This was not how she had been experiencing Jennifer. She felt she needed to let Jennifer know she was there and at least let her know she could say something if she needed to. It's like she has fainted but is still conscious, was the thought that came to mind. 'I am here if there is anything you want to tell me.' She spoke softly and gently, trying not to disturb Jennifer and interrupt whatever she might have been thinking about or feeling.

She heard Jennifer take a short, sharp breath, and then lapse back into silence. Laura waited again, straining her attention to try to hold herself as fully present and open as she could to what was happening. She could feel a tension in her body, tightening across her shoulders as she sat, slightly forward, watching and waiting. She noted that Jennifer seemed to be hardly breathing, but her eyes were open and occasionally she was blinking. The thought crossed Laura's mind that she felt she could have passed her hand in front of Jennifer's eyes and she would not have noticed.

> Jennifer is clearly engaging intensely with some kind of inner experience. How much she is actually conscious of this is unknown. Processes may be occurring within her that are outside of her awareness. But it is clearly powerful and Laura is respecting it as being something that is necessary for Jennifer at this time. The longer it goes on, the more likely it may be that Laura will want to let Jennifer know once again that she is there. But she does not want to draw Jennifer out unless she needs to – for instance, if the session is soon to end and time is needed to process the experience and help her prepare to end. Sometimes a client can be engaged in inner processes that leave them unaware of time.

Another short, sharp breath from Jennifer. And the silence continued.

Jennifer was aware of Laura, although she seemed distant yet present at the same time. She wasn't thinking of anything, and was actually just sitting. It wasn't that she was aware of feeling numb or anything, she was just sitting. She wasn't holding a sense of self that could reflect on her experiencing. She was just sitting, existing, but somehow without any self-reflective presence of thought.

Fifteen minutes had passed. Laura was resisting the fantasies that were present in her head about what might be happening. She wanted to simply stay with Jennifer. She had reminded her a number of times that she was there. She had stopped adding the 'if there was something you want to say', as clearly if there had been Jennifer would have said something.

Jennifer suddenly felt herself. She blinked and took a deep breath and looked up. She took another deep breath, lifting her hands to her face as she did so and looked over her fingertips at Laura, and then looked at the clock. She frowned. 'Is that clock right? Surely that much time hasn't elapsed, I've only just got here.'

'Yes. You have been in a long silence.'

Jennifer felt her eyes widen. 'But I've only just got here, and I remember sitting down and ... I don't understand what happened.'

'You have been sitting silently for about 15 minutes. I let you know I was here a few times, but you stayed in the silence.'

'But that can't be right, I mean, I . . . .' Jennifer thought, trying to remember something, anything. Yes, she could remember hearing Laura's voice, yes, she could remember that. 'I remember your voice.'

Laura nodded, deciding to keep with simple empathy. She wanted Jennifer to have the freedom to explore her experience without interference. 'You remember my voice.'

It is highly likely that Jennifer is in a very vulnerable and impressionable state. The need to keep empathic responses simply and directly reflective of what has been said is important. There is otherwise a high risk of the client feeling unheard or misunderstood, or of making sense of an experience based more on the therapist's perception than their own.

There is also the very real risk of the unskilled counsellor introducing material leading to accusations of inducing 'false memories'. Warner (2000, p. 170) has highlighted that 'the most important dimension of the person-centred approach for work with this clientele [those experiencing dissociation] is the attention we pay to fostering the client's symbolisation while not inserting "suggestive" material of our own'.

'I came in . . . and how did we start?' Jennifer thought back. 'Yes, something about a review. Yes, I remember you saying about a review. And then . . . .' She looked up anxiously. 'I don't remember anything else.'

'So, you remember my mentioning a review, and that's all?'

'Yes.' Jennifer shivered, although the room was not cold. 'Ooh, I don't feel good. I remember coming in feeling uncomfortable with myself. I remember wanting to tell you about it and . . . and it seems to have got lost somehow.'

'You wanted to tell me about feeling uncomfortable with yourself?'

'Yes, and I still do.' Jennifer paused, and blinked, taking another deep breath. She continued, ' I feel as though I am becoming more myself.'

'More yourself,' Laura responded, inviting Jennifer to say more with her tone of voice and again keeping her empathic response simple and direct, using Jennifer's words.

'Yes, well, strange, I mean I felt myself when I arrived, and I felt myself just now, but then there are those 15 minutes when I am not aware of feeling anything.'

'Mmmm.' Laura nodded her head gently and waited, holding her focus on Jennifer. 'In those 15 minutes not aware of feeling anything.'

Jennifer shook her head. 'It's really troubling me, and it feels like it is additional to the troubledness – is there such a word? – that I was feeling when I arrived, well, that I have been feeling on and off since I last saw you.'

'So, a sense of troubledness since I last saw you and again now after what has just occurred.'

Using the client's own word, even though it may not be a real word, often helps to convey that the client is being heard as they want to be heard. It is important not to try to turn their words into something else. Jennifer has experienced 'troubledness' so that is what Laura conveys as having heard.

'Yes, it has been really strange, and unsettling, And I can't make sense of it, I really can't.' Jennifer paused, wondering how to explain her experience. 'I have times when I seem to feel this wave of ... I can't describe it, but it kind of washes over me, no through me ....' Jennifer stopped and Laura could see she was looking puzzled and she decided to let her have the space to be with it. 'Well, it actually seems to arise within me more than anything, and it is a feeling of ... I can't describe the feeling, but it leaves me troubled, disturbed, unsettled.'

'So this feeling, this something arises within you, leaving you troubled, disturbed, unsettled, and it's within you?' Laura re-emphasised the 'within you', she wasn't sure why, but somehow it just felt important and right to do so.

'Within me, yes, as if it's in my body, low down, down here.' Jennifer pointed her hands downwards over the area beneath her solar plexus. 'And it seems to rise up and ....' She took a deep breath and closed her eyes. 'And I can feel it above my heart and ... ,' Jennifer swallowed, 'I can feel it in my throat. It's hot and hard, like gravel, yes, like hot gravel grating.'

'So you can feel it rising up,' Laura moved her hands as Jennifer had, 'and it feels hot, hard and like gravel grating in your throat?'

Jennifer nodded. 'But it's not the physical sensation as much as what I'm left feeling. It's so hard to describe.'

Laura could feel the temptation to start asking questions like: When did it happen? What are you doing or thinking about when it happens? What do you do to cope with it? She pushed them aside. Keep with the client. She is wanting to describe the experience at the moment, that is what she wants me to hear. 'The feelings are hard to describe?'

Questioning of this nature can simply take the focus out of the client's frame of reference and into the 'need to know' part of the counsellor. The person-centred counsellor keeps their focus on the client's internal world as it is being described to them, tending only to ask questions for the purpose of clarifying something that they are not sure they have heard accurately.

'I feel so unsettled by it. I know I'm not myself after it happens. It doesn't happen all the time, but it has been happening sort of regularly.'

'Not yourself afterwards and it happens sort of regularly?' Laura reflected questioningly, inviting clarification but leaving it open for Jennifer to choose which area to focus on.

'No, not at all myself. It doesn't happen when I'm at work. I guess I am more focused there. I seem to be able to get on with things and, well, it just doesn't happen. But back at home in the early evening, around the time I am eating, there it is, and it is affecting my appetite. Sometimes I don't feel like eating. I push the food around my plate. At other times, I eat fine, but not so well in the evenings. Its not every day that this happens, but it seems to be happening more frequently.'

'Happening more frequently and affecting your appetite?'

'Yeah. What is it? It's really upsetting me.' At this point Jennifer began to cry. 'My life feels so good at the moment, why is this happening to me? I hate it. I'm beginning to feel difficult about evenings. I used to look forward to coming home and spending time relaxing with Ian, or whatever, but now I find myself wondering if it will happen again tonight. I hate it, Laura, I hate it.' The tears flowed more freely as Jennifer buried her face in a tissue. After a while she took a deep breath. 'Oohh.' She shook her head.

'You feel that it is affecting you in so many ways and you hate it.'

'I don't want it to affect our relationship. I love Ian, and he's really good about it. He wants to be supportive but he doesn't know what to do. I don't know what to do.' Jennifer paused for a moment. Laura could see she was thinking, and felt it was right to give her space. 'And I've got to be honest with you, haven't I, I mean, what's the point if I'm not honest with you, and with myself? Oh God, this is difficult to say, but I'm drinking more.'

'That really was hard to say.' Laura replied wanting to empathise with this and feeling that Jennifer was aware that she had heard what she had said.

'Yeah. I hate that too. But it seems linked and I need to sort that out as well.'

'I'm wondering what you want to focus on, Jennifer?'

'I kind of feel the drinking is a reaction, and that maybe that will sort itself out if I can get to the bottom of what is happening to me.'

Laura heard what Jennifer was saying and couldn't help but wonder whether alcohol had more of a role in what was happening than Jennifer appreciated.

Jennifer has not indicated whether the alcohol use is a reaction to what she experiences, or is in some way contributing to the experience, or both. Whilst alcohol can anaesthetise feelings and is often used to quell uncomfortable feelings, for some people it can also release feelings as well, bringing them to the surface of experience (Bryant-Jefferies, 2001, 2003).

'So your feeling is that the alcohol use will take care of itself if you can resolve the experiences you are having? And I want to say that I am experiencing a wonder as to what role the alcohol actually has. This may be my own curiosity, but I am just aware of this wonder, and I don't want to take you away from what you want to focus on.'

'No that's OK. I trust your instincts. The work we did previously on my alcohol use was really helpful. Let me think. I have a glass usually before the meal, we both do, and then settle down to finish the rest of the bottle with the meal.'

'Is that always the pattern?'

'Yes, well, mostly. Sometimes I don't have the first one until we have started the meal, it depends what's going on. Sometimes Ian's home first and has cooked the meal, and then there often isn't much time before I start to eat – I have a quick shower and change, and by then it can be ready.'

Laura nodded slightly. She was aware of wondering what difference there might be between the two scenarios. 'Any difference in what you experience between these two situations?'

'Difference?' Jennifer thought for a moment. 'The difference is that . . . no, that's not right. I was going to say I drank more when I cooked, but no, that doesn't follow. No . . . .' Jennifer reflected back over the last couple of weeks. It was difficult to remember each evening. 'I'm not sure. But I think it might be interesting to keep a note of it. You remember the drinking diary I used before? Maybe I can use that to track what is happening. I kind of sense that I may be getting more uncomfortable when I cook.'

'More uncomfortable when you cook?'

Jennifer frowned. 'No, that doesn't feel right. No.' She paused and reflected back again. What did happen when she cooked? 'No, I feel more . . . , no I don't. I'm not making much sense, am I?'

'It seems really hard for you to put your experience into words that make sense to you.'

'Let me try again. When I cook I have a glass of wine, and sometimes start on a second before the meal itself.' A realisation suddenly burst upon Jennifer as she heard herself saying these words. 'Those are the times when I find it hard to eat!'

'OK, so when you drink before the meal you find it hard to eat?'

'Yes, I begin to feel uncomfortable, but what happens when I drink with the meal? I do eat better, yes, I do, but . . . .' Jennifer thought. 'But then I feel uncomfortable after the meal. Yes, it's as though the feelings are delayed.'

'As though the feelings are delayed?' Laura could feel 2 and 2 coming together in her mind to make 4 – that the alcohol was in some way inducing the discomfort, but she did not want to make this connection for Jennifer, if indeed it was the case.

'Yes, so . . . shit, it is the alcohol, isn't it? But why do I suddenly start to feel unsettled by drinking? I do feel worse when I have drunk before the meal. I often have a gin or something afterwards as well, helps me to settle again. Takes the edge off it, anyway.'

'I hear a lot of things going on here. You drink before the meal, end up feeling worse during the meal and drinking more afterwards, but when you do not drink before eating then you feel unsettled more after the meal, but it isn't so intense and you are less likely to drink more?'

Jennifer pondered on what Laura had fed back to her. 'Yes, that's it. OK. So, if I try to avoid drinking before the meal then it should be more manageable. I'll try that.'

'OK, so change the pattern a bit and see what happens, yeah?'

Laura voicing her curiosity as to the role of Jennifer's alcohol use has unwittingly directed her into a focus on this theme. A useful exploration has occurred. However, was it what Jennifer really wanted to talk about? She has, as she has said, trusted Laura's instinct, but has this cut across that important feature of the person-centred approach which encourages the client to listen to and trust their own inner prompting and evaluation of experiences?

'Yes.' Jennifer was aware of feeling quite good about what they had just been exploring, then she began to feel a shift, as if that good feeling was slowly draining away, like someone had pulled out a plug. 'There's still what happened at the start of the session today. I know we have just said that it may be something to do with the alcohol, but I'm not sure that it is only the alcohol. I mean, I don't know, I kind of feel fragile, you know, I sometimes don't feel quite right but I can't really get hold of what it is. And losing those 15 minutes at the start of the session makes me wonder if that happens at other times and I'm not aware of it? I mean, I really didn't feel as though that length of time had passed, I really didn't. It sounds crazy, but that's how it is. I feel I need to keep an eye on myself in case it does happen again. And of course there was the fainting in that previous session.' Jennifer looked at the clock, time was passing and she needed to get herself ready to end the session and head off home. She was suddenly aware of feeling quite exhausted. 'I feel really tired. I have a lot to go away and think about again.'

The session ended with Jennifer describing her tiredness and what she had ahead of her over the next couple of weeks. Laura noted the shift of focus and felt that it was probably Jennifer's way of preparing herself, given that it had been quite an intense session. They also did a short review and agreed that they would continue meeting fortnightly, and that this pattern would be disrupted in the next couple of months with holidays.

Jennifer left and Laura returned to the counselling room to sit and reflect on what had happened. That silence at the start of the session was still with her and she wondered what had been happening. She decided she would mention it at supervision, which she would be having before her next session with Jennifer. She wandered back into her kitchen, having written up her notes, and without thinking opened a bottle of wine and drank a large glass, fairly quickly. This was unusual, she rarely did this after a counselling session, and she suddenly became aware of what she had done. It left her feeling uneasy and definite that she needed a supervision session.

Supervision

Laura had been discussing two of her other clients with Malcolm, and she noticed that time had passed and she knew she wanted to spend some time talking about Jennifer. She began by briefly describing what had happened in the last two sessions, and then went on to focus on the silence and on her finding herself drinking wine after the last session.

'I really was feeling somewhat unnerved with the silence, Malcolm. It just felt, I don't know, somehow it just left me feeling uncomfortable.'

'Uncomfortable,' Malcolm reflected back, and added, 'can you say a little more about this feeling?'

Laura sat and thought for a while, trying to recapture the experience. A thought struck her which had not been present for her at the time, but now, thinking back, it seemed to somehow make sense, although she wasn't sure whether it was something that had been present or was a kind of projection backwards that she was making now on to the experience. Well, it was what had come into her mind, so she voiced it. 'This sounds really odd, and it somehow makes me feel a little cold saying it, but just now, as I was thinking back, the thought came into my mind that it was almost as if I was alone in that room. I know that's daft, I was with Jennifer and I was very aware of her sitting there in front of me, and yet ....' Laura thought again. No, surely this was something she was making up, or was it? Laura continued to try to recapture the experience of being in the room with Jennifer during that silence, and of how it had felt not knowing what was happening, what Jennifer was experiencing. 'I remember feeling that Jennifer had become distant, well, I am saying she became distant. I suppose the reality is that distance emerged between us. But it was maybe more than distance.' She stopped again, trying once more to get a feel for what had happened.

'More than distance?' was Malcolm's response, words that he spoke quietly as he sensed the delicacy of Laura's struggle to capture the subtlety of what she had experienced.

'It was as though Jennifer was not there, at least, not the Jennifer that I was used to being with, and I am really not sure at all what was present. It was as though the person I knew was not there. Of course she was there, and yet .... It really felt as though, well, I don't know.'

Malcolm nodded yet also felt a little puzzled. He wanted to clarify for himself what he thought he understood from what Laura was saying. 'So it was as though Jennifer as you knew her was not there, but you are not sure what was present, what part of her was present?' Malcolm deliberately used the word 'part'. It seemed to him that the aspect of Jennifer that was known to Laura had temporarily taken a back seat and allowed something else to emerge.

'Do I mean another part?' Laura thought about it. 'Yes, I suppose I do, but I cannot define this part. It ... well, I mean, it sort of didn't have any substance and yet ...,' Laura thought again, 'and yet something was present because I can still remember the intensity. But somehow Jennifer seemed to look kind of blank. I remember thinking, yes that's right, I remember thinking I could pass my hand in front of her eyes and she wouldn't have seen it.'

'Sounds to me as though she dissociated into a place in herself from which she was unable to communicate, a place from which she ....' A phrase had come into Malcolm's mind from somewhere and it felt strong. 'A place where she had, or should I say has, no voice.'

The dissociative state alluded to here could be the presence within Jennifer of a part of herself that had no voice during a traumatic episode in the past, and which continues to have no voice. This could have emerged because what was experienced was too distressing and was pushed away and not allowed a voice, for to have that voice would have left Jennifer flooded by painful and unbearable feelings. Another possibility is that one part of Jennifer is stopping another part from speaking. During the silence a kind of internal psychological censorship may have occurred, leaving Jennifer unable to say anything about the discomfort she had been experiencing. The fact, as well, that she lost all sense of time is indicative that a dissociative state may have emerged.

'No voice. Yet somehow it wasn't as if Jennifer had a sense of wanting to say something. She couldn't remember anything about the experience. She really had slipped into another place in herself.' Laura suddenly found herself thinking back to that earlier session when Jennifer had fainted. 'Do you remember the session when she fainted? There was something around about feeling paralysed. I can't remember exactly what happened, but she said something about feeling paralysed, of being aware of feeling that way but being unable to communicate it in words.'

'Paralysed with no voice. Distant. And you felt uncomfortable.' Malcolm offered back what he felt to be key elements to what Laura had been saying.

'Yes, I felt uncomfortable and I felt the distance. But I am stuck with this notion of being paralysed with no voice. It was more than vocal paralysis. I mean, her body hardly moved throughout the silence. She blinked occasionally, and took a deep breath now and then, but otherwise, well, she just wasn't moving. But she hadn't passed out, her eyes were open, but ..., but there was, well, nothing. I don't know what to make of it but I know it is significant, and it is happening now. I've been seeing Jennifer for a year now, and nothing like this has happened before. Why now? Something is going on, something is coming to the surface, but it cannot tell me anything yet. I know I have to stay with it, and allow whatever is present to reveal itself, at least, if I can offer sufficient unconditional positive regard so that it feels safe to do so.'

'I think you are right. Something is perhaps emerging from deep within Jennifer, and it is fragile, and it is struggling to find a voice, and it may almost need coaxing but gently, very gently. Don't forget there may be other parts of her working against this emergence, and they must also feel unconditional positive regard and not feel threatened.'

Malcolm recognised that as a supervisor he had a kind of educational role, drawing attention to aspects of the counselling work that his supervisees may not have noted. It reminded him of a phrase he had read some years back: 'A good supervisor is ideally a teacher, a conscience, a friend and more – knowing when to support and when to push' (Williams, 1992, p. 440). He sensed as well Laura's need to feel supported.

'Yes, I need to be aware of that. You're right, thanks for reminding me. It is easy to get carried away with wanting to hear the voiceless part and forget that there may be another part that is seeking to maintain the voicelessness, but which also needs attending to. And I have to let it happen at its own pace. I know I cannot push it. I trust that Jennifer's process is actively causing something to emerge, and I must stay with it.' Laura suddenly remembered something, 'And it would start happening just as we are approaching the summer break. Jennifer is due to have a couple of weeks away and then I am away for most of August. There is going to be about a five-week break after the next session, and whilst I know Jennifer is aware of this, and I can sit here and say that I trust her process, I am anxious about whether she may be able to contain it. I mean, I don't want to leap to conclusions here, but if we are looking at a dissociative process then there may not simply be a lone voice seeking to communicate something that happened in her past.'

'It is a big leap of assumption and yet it is perhaps a reasonable one to make, although we cannot be sure. Sometimes speculation can run away with us, and take us away from the reality of what is being experienced by the client and by us in relationship with them. And yet, at the same time, it can be helpful to reflect on these matters to inform our understanding of what *may* be occuring.'

'I guess I am jumping ahead here, but my concern is that if there is a dissociative process within her self-structure, then there could be elements that are destructive, and elements that simply may not experience time or are unaware of the implications of a break in therapy.'

Malcolm nodded. 'We cannot be sure, it is an assumption, and yet we cannot ignore the possibility. And it *is* really leaving you anxious, isn't it?'

Laura nodded. 'I do trust her process but I also cannot deny my anxiety in all of this.'

Malcolm could really sense the anxiety that Laura was experiencing, she was sitting in a tighter posture and clearly she needed support and reassurance. He noted that he felt anxious for her. 'I guess I am parallel processing here in that I am feeling anxiety for you whilst also wanting to trust your process in handling this. You're a good therapist, Laura, and you need to take breaks from counselling. The client is aware that the break in counselling is coming up but nevertheless her process has chosen this time to push memories to the surface.'

'Parallel processing' here refers to a process in which the supervisor is experiencing feelings, thoughts, or even may act out something in relation to the supervisee that is also present for the supervisee in her relationship with her client. It could simply be that what is present within the supervisor (their own material/process) has a certain resonance with that which is present for the supervisee. This will need to be clarified. However, it can be an indicator of the potency of the material or experiencing that is being processed in parallel between them, signifying a need for further exploration as to its nature and effect on both the counselling and supervision process. The self-awareness of the supervisor that informs their congruence should enable them to distinguish the origin of what has become present for them.

'I am just so aware of the complexity of it all and wondering whether Jennifer can contain it.'
'Yes, it is complex, and you say "contain *it*"?' Malcolm was curious what meaning Laura might be attaching to 'it'.
'Well, whatever it is may be emerging, whatever it is that has not got a voice. It could happen anytime, couldn't it? I mean, it may not conveniently happen before or during a therapy session.'

Whilst this is true, it is also worth considering that what may be currently hidden from Jennifer's awareness may need the empathic understanding and warm acceptance offered within a therapy session to feel able to emerge. Perhaps, therefore, her process can be trusted and the voiceless part will seek an appropriately supportive moment to emerge.

Malcolm could sense Laura's very real concern, and he shared it too, although he was also aware that he wanted to feel able to trust that whatever did emerge into Jennifer's awareness would emerge at a time when she would be in a place to manage it. 'You know, it may be that for those parts of herself to emerge she may actually need the experience of empathy and warm acceptance to be present. It could be that without the right therapeutic environment they will remain hidden away. But we cannot be sure. I really sense your concern and I want to ask you what would make you feel more at ease.'
'Well, I guess I'd like to feel that Jennifer has a named person she can contact if she needs to, you know, if something does happen and she needs to talk it through, even if only over the phone. I think I would feel more at ease, and I think there is some professional responsibility here.' They discussed it and Malcolm agreed to act as cover.

A supervisor will already have insight into the client's issues and process and so from that perspective could be regarded as a positive choice. However, this could be conveyed to another counsellor. From the client's perspective, they will already be aware that their counsellor's work with them is discussed in supervision and they may feel comfortable that the cloak of confidentiality is being maintained within known boundaries, rather than extended outwards to include another counsellor and, potentially, their supervisor as well. However, if Malcolm is suggested and contacted, the client will then have formed a direct relationship with him which may have consequences for her attitude towards Laura. I have myself experienced this situation as a supervisor covering for supervisees and have only been contacted once, and it was a minimal contact that did not seem to have any unhealthy impact on the client, their relationship with their counsellor, or their counsellor's relationship with me. However, it is something to be thought through on a case-by-case basis, and would require open and frank discussion with the client.

Malcolm highlighted the issue of raising this with Jennifer. 'I am also wondering how you might introduce the idea without, well, without almost encouraging greater anxiety in Jennifer, or maybe even some curiosity about me, which is probably unavoidable.'

'Hmm, good point. I want to be real with Jennifer, so I could say that as she has been having some intense experiences, would she like a phone number of someone to contact should she feel she needed to?' Laura frowned, 'But then I really would be conveying something about not trusting her to handle things, and that could be detrimental, couldn't it? I'm also not sure whether I can pre-plan it anyway. Maybe I should hold this in my awareness and see how the next session goes. I really would like to feel that she asks if she feels she needs to. I realise part of my motivation for all of this is my own peace of mind, but not wholly so. It was the intensity of that silence. I just think it would be . . . , well, I was going to say almost abusive, given the situation, not to offer something.'

'So you want to offer her something both personally and professionally, but you don't want to undermine her?'

'Yes. I need to see how the session goes and see how I might introduce it in the context of discussing the break in counselling. Yes, that seems best, to discuss the break during the next session and ask her if she feels she would like anyone to contact should the need arise. She knows I have a supervisor and it would mean not getting someone else involved.'

'OK, we'll go with that. But can you let me know whether you have given her my number as I guess I won't be seeing you again until after you come back.'

Laura agreed to do this, and then moved the discussion on to her experience of drinking that large glass of wine after the last session. What emerged from the exploration was that it was clearly out of character and that Laura had been almost in another place in herself. Whilst she had been aware of what she was doing, she was not really engaging any thought about it. It was as though she had been on automatic pilot. 'I really had picked something up, or something in me had been somehow affected by Jennifer. I need to be aware of this. I do wonder at the impact our clients can have on us, particularly when they enter into these deeper states. And it makes me think about my own drinking, not that I drink much now, but in the past, I guess I have used it to unwind, to affect how I feel, I'm sure I have, that's why most of us drink, isn't it?'

Malcolm had nodded, and commented that in his experience it sometimes seemed as though, where a deep connection was established, the counsellor could find themselves behaving in ways that were unexpected and out of character for them, yet perfectly in character for their client. 'I don't think we fully understand the mechanism and the processes associated with connecting at depth with people who are reliving experiences from their past in an immediate way. But I think that the empathic connection we establish can go beyond empathy, and something far more profound happens, creating some kind of resonance with us, or maybe part of us, which has its own associated behaviours. Makes me aware of how vital it is to work on our congruence, on our own self-awareness and to be able to recognise these kinds of reactions and, where necessary, resolve them in therapy.'

'Yes, and whilst it initially unnerved me, I also smiled and recognised that in a sense Jennifer had got to me. I remember thinking of it that way. Perhaps we connect in ways beyond our conscious awareness? These things are so immeasurable it is hard to understand.'

The supervision session drew to a close with both Malcolm and Laura agreeing that in the science (or is it an art?) of human relationship, therapy was perhaps only beginning to grope blindly towards a real understanding of what it was.

Points for discussion

- Did you feel that Laura responded in a person-centred way to both the fainting attack and the silence? What leads you to your conclusion?
- How do you react to Jennifer wanting to extend the time between sessions? Would you have responded differently, and how would your response relate to person-centred principles?
- Was it therapeutically helpful for Laura to express her curiosity regarding Jennifer's alcohol use?
- What are your experiences of dissociative states or working with them in a client? If the idea is new to you, what feelings and thoughts does this explanation of client-experiencing evoke in you?
- Working with silence can be challenging. What impact does a lengthy silence with a client have on maintaining empathy?

- Given that you have now read more of the counselling sessions, review your thoughts as to what is happening for Jennifer in terms of person-centred theory.
- Evaluate Laura's offering of the core conditions within the counselling sessions in this chapter.
- Did you feel that Malcolm offered Laura what was needed in her supervision session both for her and for her client?

CHAPTER 4

Counselling session 36

It was 7.35pm and Jennifer had not yet arrived. The rain was streaming down the windows and Laura could hear the gutters beginning to overflow. Not a nice night to be out, she thought, and wondered whether there had been any flooding on the roads nearby. She saw Jennifer's car drawing up and she went out to the door so she could let her straight in.

'Sorry I'm late. It's awful out there.'

'Yes, not a nice night to be out. Come on in. Here, let me take your coat and umbrella. Go on through and I'll be with you in a moment.'

'Thanks.' Jennifer went into Laura's counselling room. She had had a couple of disturbing weeks again, more so than before, and had had some strange images from her past that she could not really make sense of. She was aware of feeling very anxious about the forthcoming session given what had happened in recent sessions. But she also felt she needed to persevere. She didn't want to hold back, she wanted to understand herself.

Laura came in and smiled. 'So, where do you want to start this evening?' Laura wanted to keep it open so that Jennifer could take her own direction.

Jennifer responded, looking deep into Laura's eyes. 'I'm feeling disturbed again, and more so. And I don't understand.'

'More disturbed than before and you don't understand.' Laura noticed the anxious look in Jennifer's eyes and added, 'And you look anxious.'

'Yes. But I'm not sure where to start.' Jennifer sat and thought. She had been wondering where to begin on the journey over. The drinking? That had got worse. The discomfort? That had increased, particularly during the evenings. The disturbed sleep? That had become an annoying routine.

Laura sensed that Jennifer was having trouble trying to decide where to start. She didn't want to stop her process so she left Jennifer with her thoughts.

'Well, I suppose it is this feeling of being so unsettled, particularly in the evening, but I'm waking up in the night, with my heart thumping, my chest tight, and sweating. And it takes me a long while to settle back down and get back to sleep. I invariably have to get up, have a glass of water and sit in the front room for a bit, partly to cool down, but somehow I need to get out of the bedroom. I don't know why. It's not every night, but most nights.'

'Mmmm. Most nights.' Laura didn't want to say much but rather to leave Jennifer to continue as she was in more of a 'talking about' mode rather than expressing feelings present in the here and now.

This distinction can be quite helpful when deciding the nature of an empathic response. Often where the client is talking about what has been happening, then acknowledging what has been said by reflecting the last things said can be enough. This is not appropriate or helpful, however, where the client is expressing deep thoughts and feelings present in the moment, where accurate empathic responses are required, generally using the client's word, to ensure that the client does feel heard and that what they are seeking to convey is being understood, and is warmly accepted as the client's reality.

'Yes. And it seems to be mainly on nights when I have drunk a little more, but not every time. So I don't think it's the drink. I tried to reduce, and some nights I have, but mostly it has gone up. I just feel this kind of creeping anxiety starting to come over me when I get home from work. There's nothing I am thinking about to make me feel like that, but once I start I then begin to worry about other things: work, my relationship with Ian, will we have children, what to cook, what to buy when I'm next out shopping, have I got enough soap powder, all kinds of things start to flood my brain. I have an extra glass or two of wine to shut it down.' She shook her head. 'And then I have these awful episodes in the night. I wake up feeling as though I can't breathe, my chest is so tight. Feels like a weight on me.'

Laura nodded and thought for a moment. Should she hold Jennifer on this experience of weight and see what emerged? She decided not to, but rather to reflect Jennifer's words so as not to introduce anything else. 'You can't breathe, your chest is tight, feels like a weight on you.'

'Yes, real heavy.'

'Real heavy.' Laura spoke slowly, sensing that this was leading Jennifer more deeply into her experience.

Jennifer took a deep breath and closed her eyes. She took another deep breath and opened them again. 'Yes, and I feel so hot. Like I'm burning up.' She shook her head. 'I don't know what it is about. It really disturbs me, and these broken nights are leaving me feeling tired and irritable, and that doesn't help. I thought about going to the doctor to get some sleeping tablets, but I'd rather not, well not yet anyway. I hope it's some kind of phase and I'll come out of it. But I really do want to get back to being me again. I don't feel like myself, I really don't. I just feel so on edge.'

Laura could feel a wave of tiredness coming over her. 'Don't feel yourself, feeling so on edge. It feels really heavy, and really tiring.' She hadn't planned to say the last three words, but they kind of came out. She was feeling tired and heavy herself and somehow it felt relevant to what she had heard Jennifer say, although she had only talked about heaviness.

Laura hasn't really owned the tiredness and heaviness, Jennifer has interpreted it as an empathic response to what she had said and is feeling. Sometimes this can happen, the counsellor congruently saying something expressive of what they are feeling but because it is so present for the client they experience it as an empathic response.

'Yes, very tired and everything seems such an effort at the moment. I don't seem to be enjoying anything. I don't know. Do you think it's the alcohol?'

'You wonder if the extra alcohol is doing it?'

'Well, yes, but then I kind of know that it isn't really that. I'm sure it doesn't help although it feels like it does in the evening. I don't know. I guess I feel all confused over everything.'

'Yeah, I really do sense your confusion. I can see it in your eyes, it just feels very present.'

'And it's scary too. I mean, what's happening to me?' Laura noticed a tear bubble out of Jennifer's right eye and trickle down her cheek. She closed her eyes, opened them and more tears flowed out of both eyes. She reached for a tissue.

'Scary, very scary, wondering what is happening, what is happening to you.'

Jennifer closed her eyes again. 'I really don't want to go back to drinking so heavily again. It seems to help me settle back down but it doesn't really, it just takes the edge off it. And then in the morning I feel tired and irritable. I feel edgy but it is different to the evenings somehow. It's hard to explain. But it is different.' Jennifer stopped and thought for a moment. 'It feels more unnerving in the evenings.'

'Irritable and edgy in the mornings and more unnerving in the evenings.' Laura was not aware that she had emphasised 'evenings' as she spoke.

Laura has unwittingly directed Jennifer to a focus on the evenings. However much the person-centred counsellor tries to avoid directing the client, it can still happen. Where it is noted it can be explored in supervision. In this case, Laura has missed it. Maintaining a non-directive attitude is extremely challenging and requires a lot of focus and concentration. So often the directive element can creep in not so much through what is said as through how it is said. There is a necessary discipline to person-centred working.

'Yes, there is something about when I get home and I am waiting for Ian to get back, usually between 6.00pm and 7.00pm. That hour can feel like an eternity. I can't settle. You know, I've cut myself a couple of times preparing the dinner this last week. That's not me. I'm usually much too careful.'

Laura was listening intently and feeling increasingly anxious herself, wondering how powerful whatever was unsettling Jennifer was. She wanted to maintain her empathy and warmth for Jennifer, and she was aware of experiencing a heightened sense of her own self, which had kind of emerged as she had witnessed Jennifer's tears.

'So something just doesn't feel right somehow, doesn't feel like you?'

The cuts may well be accidental, innocent lapses in concentration, or could they be a self-abusing dissociated part emerging? Jennifer's talking of not feeling herself.

Jennifer lapsed into silence. No, she thought, this isn't me, this really isn't me.

'Feels like I'm going mad, sometimes. Am I going mad?'

'I don't think so, but it is something you wonder about.'

'I do. Where's it coming from?' Jennifer blew the air out through her nose. 'Well, I guess it can only be coming from me! But . . . oh, I don't know. It all feels like such an effort. And look at that rain. Will it ever stop?' She looked out of the window. As she did so she felt something shifting inside her. The window began to change shape. It wasn't the window in Laura's room anymore. It was familiar though. The net curtains were different yet she recognised the pattern of tiny flowers. And she could see the curtains on either side. They were the ones her mother had in the lounge where they lived when she was a girl, well, when she was – how old was she? When she was about 7. The window seemed bigger though. And she felt strangely smaller. She could feel tears in her eyes and fear in her stomach, real fear, tight, hot, churning. She felt sick with it. And then it passed. She closed her eyes and when she opened them she was back in Laura's room, and feeling herself again. That strange smallness had passed.

'Oh, that was weird.' Her mouth was dry. She reached out and sipped from the glass of water that was always available on the side table.

'Weird?' Laura wasn't sure what had happened. It had just seemed to her that Jennifer had lost herself momentarily looking out of the window.

'I . . . oh this is silly.'

'What's silly Jennifer?'

'Yes, well, I mean. Oh I don't know. For a minute there I felt as though I was back in the house where I lived as a child.'

Laura nodded. 'Mmmm.'

'It was as though I was looking out of the lounge window. It was late afternoon.' Jennifer looked startled. 'I don't know why I said that. I hadn't thought of that but somehow I know it was in the afternoon.'

Laura was giving Jennifer her full attention, focusing her senses to absorb what she was saying.

'I was looking out of the window and it was raining, like it is now. And I remember the net curtains, they had little flowers on them. I used to count them as a child, and look at the patterns and the way each flower connected to the rest of the pattern. It was, and is, so vivid. Like it was yesterday. No, closer than yesterday, like it was there a moment ago. Ooh,' Jennifer shivered 'that feels really peculiar. But it is, was, no *is* so vivid. And as I sat looking out of the window. No, no I wasn't sitting. I must have been kneeling, yes, I used to kneel and lean on the back of the chair. And my stomach was churning. I felt fear, so much fear, and I was crying, but silently. There was no one there to hear my cries. But I don't know why I was crying. But I was hurting inside.'

Jennifer had stopped speaking and Laura quietly reflected back on what she had last said. 'So much hurt inside.' Laura wondered whether that might have sounded patronising but she wanted to let Jennifer know she had heard her but did not want to say anything lengthy and disturb her flow.

Tears were rolling down Jennifer's cheeks again. 'I can feel the hurt now.'

'Mmmm.' Laura did not want to disturb what Jennifer was feeling.

Jennifer continued to cry. She could feel emotions welling up inside of herself, and she could feel that there was fear present, real fear. More than fear. It felt more like terror, but she did not know why. The feeling kept coming and the tears would not stop. Slowly, the feeling began to ease but she still felt very raw inside. Somehow those curtains kept coming back to her, and the sensation of terror. She shivered and took a deep breath, blowing the air back out of her mouth. 'What was that about? It felt, feels, so real. But I don't understand why. I feel very, very on edge at the moment.' She took a tissue and dried her face, then reached over to the glass and took some sips of water. Her mouth had gone dry.

'You really have no idea what the feelings were about but that terror was/is very present.'

Jennifer shook her head and found herself instinctively turning again to the window. 'It's like I know something but I don't know it, like I have a sense of something but I cannot get hold of what it is.'

'Something but can't get hold of it.' Laura kept to a brief response, holding an empathic focus and allowing Jennifer freedom to follow where her own process took her. She was aware of her own thought processes wanting to take her into her own world of speculation, but pushed that aside. She needed to be very clear and responsive to Jennifer as she struggled to make sense of her experience.

'It's like having feelings but they don't seem to be attached to anything. It's really unnerving. Really unnerving. I don't like it at all.' Jennifer paused and added, 'I feel very uncertain about myself. I feel small, I feel ... I just feel very, very small.' She looked up at Laura and looked deeply into her eyes.

'Very, very small,' Laura replied slowly, consciously aware that she was speaking quietly and slowly and sensing that perhaps Jennifer was about to connect again with childhood memories and experiences.

Silence. And it felt very silent. Laura again felt her perspective shifting as she sensed Jennifer reconnecting with her own past.

'I'm afraid.' The voice was quiet and timid, not Jennifer's usual voice.

'Afraid.'

Laura does not ask what Jennifer is afraid of. She knows that this is likely to be a very sensitive moment for Jennifer. Perhaps a voice from her childhood is seeking to be heard, and it will need to be listened to gently and sensitively. Anything disturbing or too threatening might cause it to retreat and maybe a therapeutic opportunity will be lost.

'So afraid, but I can't tell you what about. It's a secret.'

'A secret,' Laura paused, and added, 'that you can't tell me about.'

'No. I mustn't.'

'You mustn't tell me.' Laura noted to herself that 'can't' had become 'mustn't', a very different meaning. But she also recognised the voice she was listening to could very likely feel threatened by being pushed into clarifying this. It was not appropriate. She needed to allow this part of Jennifer to speak, to be attentive to it, to offer it warmth, experiences that it may never have had.

'No. I promised.'

'You promised.'

Laura does not ask who the promise was made to, again sensing that this question could be threatening and cause this part of Jennifer to retreat. There can be a temptation to want to push and find out, but in reality the client's own process must be trusted. It is likely that the voice now emerging has not spoken in years, perhaps never before. Therapy at this depth takes time and the client dictates the time. This kind of issue cannot be hurried or attempted to be resolved within a time-limited framework.

There was a pause. 'I'd like to tell you, but ... but I'd better not 'cos I'd be sure to get into trouble. And I don't want to get into trouble.' Jennifer was shaking her head as she spoke.

'You don't want to get into trouble, do you?'

'No, I don't.'

Silence again. Laura felt a strong urge to ask Jennifer her age. She thought about it, wondering whether this would be therapeutically helpful, or whether it was just her own curiosity. No, it might be helpful to have an idea of her age, and she can always refuse to tell me.

'So, how old are you, Jennifer?'

'7, but I'm nearly 8.'

'7, but nearly 8.' Laura smiled gently. 'Do you know my name?'

'Yes, you're Laura, and I like you.' Silence again. 'But I feel very alone.'

'Very alone?'

'No one to talk to, not to *really* talk to.' Laura noticed how much emphasis Jennifer had placed on 'really'. She responded with similar emphasis.

'No one to *really* talk to.'

'No.' She said the word quite sharply, and her face looked very sad as she said it.

'And it's very lonely with no one to really talk to.'

'Yes.' Jennifer's facial expression changed. It visibly brightened. 'But I do other things as well. I play with my dolls and I have got three big ones.'

'Three big dolls,' Laura replied, 'and have they got names?'

> The counsellor seeks to engage with the 7-year-old part of Jennifer by showing interest in what she is being told. She keeps her language simple. Some parts can be very dissociated to the point of being quite independent, and when this arises the counsellor really has to build a new relationship with this part. She needs to earn the 7-year-old's trust. She needs to demonstrate that she is prepared to listen and warmly accept her and be genuine to her. This may already be experienced, known and trusted by the Jennifer that Laura has been working with, but not by the 7-year-old part for which this is all new.

'Yes. One's called Lucy, she's pretty and has black hair. And there's Mandy, she's got blonde hair and big blue eyes. And there's Annabelle. She's my favourite. She has lots of nice clothes and I play with her most.'

'Lucy, Mandy and Annabelle, and you like Annabelle most. Why do you like Annabelle most Jennifer?'

'Because she's like me and she needs to be cared for. And I can dress her up.'

'Annabelle's like you and needs to be cared for, and you like dressing her up.'

'Yes.' Jennifer's facial expression began to change. It started to take on a much more serious expression. Laura sensed a shift taking place. 'I've got to go now.' And with that she had gone, and she was looking at Jennifer who was blinking and looking very bemused.

'What happened?'

'Were you aware of what was happening?'

> Sometimes a client may be aware of what a part of them is voicing during this kind of experience, at other times they may have dissociated to the point of being unaware of what is being said. Where there is no memory of what is being said and the client wants to know, then the counsellor must be very careful in ensuring accuracy and not speculating on anything or drawing any conclusions. The possibility of implanting ideas, memories and interpretations is very real and must be avoided. The transition from one dissociated part to another, or back to the usual person, can be abrupt. Warner (2000) refers to this as *switching* and comments on how clients very often cannot remember what has happened during the period in which the dissociated part has taken over their consciousness and awareness. In this case, however, Jennifer is aware but cannot intervene, she can only listen.

'Yes, I heard myself speaking, but I couldn't do anything except listen. It was really odd. But it was me. I did have three dolls and those were their names. I haven't thought about them in ages. That really was me talking, wasn't it?'

'Was that how you experienced what happened just now?' Laura did not want to confirm anything, but rather to allow Jennifer to reach her own conclusion.

'Yes. Me at 7. But I was holding back, wasn't I? I was holding something back. I couldn't tell you something, and I don't know what that was. I had no sense of what I was not saying, well, when I say I, I mean, the . . . I don't know what I mean. But that was me, wasn't it? But my voice, it seemed so timid and unsure at first.'

'Was that how you were from your memory now as an adult as you look back to your childhood?' Laura asked the question and immediately wondered whether it was helpful as it was taking Jennifer away from her feelings about what had just occurred.

'I was quite a moody and irritable child. I think I was a real pain in many ways. I didn't really do that well at school, I kind of messed around a bit. I never really seemed to be able to settle much, I don't know why.'

'Moody, irritable, messed around, found it hard to settle, yeah?'

'Yes. I mean, I had a happy childhood.' Jennifer's voice trailed off as she said this. She frowned and looked puzzled, and thoughtful. She looked at Laura searchingly. She felt suddenly uncomfortable. Yes, she had had a happy childhood, that's what she always told people, and that's what she felt and remembered. The window caught her attention, and it was still raining outside. But why had she been so unhappy? She felt herself drift into her own thoughts. She had been happy, she couldn't remember not being happy. But she had been terrified a little while ago when she remembered looking through the window as a little girl. But she had been happy. She *had* been happy. She had had a happy childhood. Her mind was beginning to race. She had to have had a happy childhood. She had to. The thoughts raced faster and faster. She *was* a happy child. She *was*. She *was*. She burst into tears, sobbing and feeling the tears hot in her eyes.

Jennifer has created an image of childhood for herself probably to enable her to feel comfortable with herself. The idea of having had a happy childhood is a compelling one, and is likely to feel more satisfying for people to hold on to. Perhaps she learned that people should have a happy childhood and this became, for her, what is termed in person-centred theory as an 'introject' which she then needed to maintain, at least in her own mind and heart, even though it may not have been her experienced reality. Another possibility here is that it may have been at least in part generated as a reflex against the terror that Jennifer has mentioned, a terror that currently remains linked to memories that are beyond her conscious awareness as an adult.

Jennifer has entered into an important stage. Her view of her childhood has been challenged, not by someone else but by herself, by the 7-year-old voice from her childhood that is trying to say that all was not well.

'I feel terrible,' were the words that Jennifer finally managed to say through the sobs. 'I feel as though I have been torn apart inside myself. I feel raw, absolutely raw, and scared, so very scared.' The sobbing increased again. Laura was aware of not only concentrating in her head on what was happening, but she was also seeking to be open to the flow of feelings within herself. Raw, scared, torn apart, these words remained with her as she witnessed Jennifer's anguish. A large part of her world has just fallen apart, she thought to herself. She recognised that she had not got the faintest idea what would happen next. The temptation was to try to think ahead, but she knew that would take her away from Jennifer. She let her know that she had heard what she had said.

'Torn apart, raw and very, very scared.'

Jennifer nodded and continued to sob. She still felt terrible inside, yet she also began to sense feeling different in some way, although she could not quite define what the difference was. She took a deep breath and could feel the pressure inside herself beginning to subside. A couple more tissues later and Jennifer looked up again. 'Oh God. I think I have been carrying around a false view of my childhood. Now I don't know what to think, what to believe. I feel like I'm in limbo, in a kind of "not-knowing" state. It's like I'm not where I was but I don't know where I am.' Jennifer paused. Her face looked very serious. 'No, it's worse than that. No, it's not that I don't know where I am, it's . . . I don't think I know *who* I am.'

Laura nodded, and repeated back slowly word for word what Jennifer had just said, 'I don't think I know *who* I am', and with the same emphasis.

Jennifer sat and just shook her head. She was now feeling strangely numb, and empty inside. A short while ago her head had been racing, now it seemed to have stopped and it was hard to think about anything. She just felt, well, in limbo.

'I really don't. Yet I know that I do as well. But somehow I don't at the same time. Am I making any sense because I'm really not sure that I am?'

'I hear you saying that whilst in one sense you do not know who you are, another part of you is saying that you do. And both seem to be happening together?'

'That's the weird bit. I know who I am but . . . .' Jennifer sat and thought about it.

Laura had a strong sense of how much thinking Jennifer was doing and she felt a strong sense that she was split between her thinking and her feeling, and that she could not think her way into her feelings.

'I'm not sure if this is helpful, but I have a strong sense of how you may be thinking that you know yourself but *feeling* that you don't.'

'Yes.' The word came out immediately as Laura finished speaking. 'Yes. And I thought I had had a happy childhood. I think I had felt that I had as well. But now I feel different and it is forcing me to think differently. But it is hard. I don't know what to think and I don't know what to feel about the past.'

Jennifer is openly confronting herself. She is no longer siding with her 'should have a happy childhood' introject. She realises *for herself*, and this is important, that things were maybe not as she has believed for so long.

It is an example of just how challenging to the client working in a person-centred way can be. But the uniqueness of the person-centred approach is that the client is offered the space to challenge themselves when they feel ready and able to do this, not through the therapist forcing them to confront some apparent inconsistency.

Jennifer rested her forehead in her hand. 'Shit. I've got a hell of a lot to think about, Laura, and I don't know where to start. What a time for this to all erupt, just before I go off on holiday.'

'That must leave you with all kinds of thoughts and feelings.' Laura deliberately responded in this general and open way, not sure whether Jennifer wanted to stay with her feeling and thoughts about childhood, or begin to think through how she might deal with the next few weeks.

'I am aware that we won't be having any sessions for a while, and I am wondering ... I was going to say, wondering how I would cope. But at the moment that seems a long way off. I'm not really sure what I am wondering about having to cope with. But I know that we won't be able to meet up again until later in August and that's about six weeks away. I'm really not too sure how I will be feeling after the holiday. I hope it will be what I need, a chance to relax, get some sun and generally take life easy. The Greek Islands are good for that and I just want to chill out.'

'What do you think would help you?' Laura was aware of the discussion she had had with her supervisor about cover when she was away, but she did not want to introduce this, but rather she wanted Jennifer to define for herself what she felt her needs might be and how they might be addressed.

Jennifer thought for a moment, but not for long. 'I guess it would be good to have someone with whom I could get in touch if I needed to.'

'OK. So the idea of someone to get in touch with if you needed to.'

'Yes, I think I'd somehow feel a little more secure in some way, for the time when I'm back and you are away. When I'm away myself, well, I can't do much about that, but maybe being away from everything will help things settle down a bit.'

'So you sense you would feel more secure when you're back and hope things will settle when you are away.'

'Yes, but I'm not sure I want to have to start going through everything with someone else. So I feel a bit stuck.'

'I was just wondering whether it could be anyone or someone who had an appreciation of what you are experiencing at the moment?'

'The latter, definitely. I think to try and explain all of this to someone else, they'd think I was mad.' Jennifer smiled. 'Have you a clone you can leave behind?'

'Nice idea, but no. Look, how would you feel about my giving you the phone number of my supervisor? We did in fact discuss whether he would be prepared to take any calls from any of my clients who might need support. I will be seeing him again before you return from holiday and can bring him up to date, if you think that would be helpful.'

Jennifer thought for a moment and was very aware of feeling a sense of relief. 'Yes. But only if I really needed to call. I think from where I am at the moment it is the knowing that there is someone I can call. I probably won't, but knowing it does make me feel less anxious. When you suggested it I felt a sense of relief.'

The session drew to a close with Laura giving Jennifer Malcolm's name and number. She still felt that Jennifer was only just beginning to get a sense of her childhood, that clearly there were events and experiences that had not yet come to light, but there were clear signs that something was being kept 'secret', the word that Jennifer in her 7-year-old state had used. But she also trusted that Jennifer's own process as a person would seek to keep her safe, and maybe memories would not surface until the counselling continued next month. But she saw no harm in having a contingency plan by way of Malcolm's number if required.

Jennifer left the session in a very pensive mood. She knew she felt different, lighter somehow, and a little unburdened in some way. But she also knew that she carried a sense of feeling distinctly uneasy. She was glad she had the holiday ahead of her, and she felt that this would do her good. She had Malcolm's number in her pocket if she needed it when she got back, and that felt reassuring. The rain had eased a little as she pulled away from in front of Laura's house. It was still light and she could see an edge to the clouds in the west. She hoped that maybe there was an edge on the horizon to the clouds within herself.

Supervision

'Before I say anything about any of my other clients, I do want to mention Jennifer. I gave her your number as we agreed, and she was very grateful. I have only seen her once since our last session, she is currently on holiday and due back next week. I want to bring you up to date with the last session.'

'Fine. What's been happening and how are you with the process?'

'In the last session Jennifer twice slipped back into a place in herself that was very much part of her childhood. Firstly, she was looking out of the window and said that the window changed to the one she remembered looking out of as a child, and of feeling fear, in fact I think she used the word terror. She had been talking about the evenings and waiting for her partner, Ian, to come home. That's a difficult time for her, and she does often drink wine at that time. Oh, and she talked about having disturbed nights, waking up sweaty and uneasy and having to go to another room to calm down. But the window experience seemed to touch some depth. It really seemed to have taken her back, and she talked of being fearful as she looked out, as if she was anticipating something, but she couldn't get hold of what it was.'

'How was that for you?'

'It felt very profound, and very real, and it drew me into a heightened sense of focus. I did have a sense of Jennifer shifting. The silence was intense. It didn't last very long, but it clearly had a powerful effect, and I am sure it was a kind of precursor to what happened later in the session.'

'A powerful effect and then something else happened?'

'Jennifer suddenly started to get very small on me, you know, a shift of perspective, and then she began to speak but this time her voice was like a little girl. She was timid and said she had a secret that she couldn't tell me. She said she knew who I was. I asked her age, but I didn't push her on the secret. I didn't want her to back away. It seemed right to keep it gentle and non-invasive.'

Malcolm nodded. 'Yes, I think you were very wise. That part of her needs to feel safe with you in order to find its voice in your presence.' He well recognised the need for a slowly, slowly, softly, softly approach.

'Well, she spoke for a while, then flipped into talking about her three dolls – what were they – Lucy, Mandy and Annabelle, and then announced that she had to go. With that she kind of faded and Jennifer in her adult state returned, blinking and bemused, but aware of the conversation that I had had with her child-self, or whatever we should call that part of her that spoke.'

Laura has neglected to remember that Annabelle was the favourite and why. This could be a lapse of memory, but it could be that Laura did not really hear this part, and may indicate that there is something from her own past blocking her.

Unless Malcolm experiences a sense of something important being unsaid, it is unlikely that he will pick up on this. The supervisor needs to be both empathically sensitive and also highly sensitive to his own responses. Offering supervision in a person-centred way requires a somewhat disciplined ability to be open in two directions at the same time as well as attempting to be open to the possibility that things are not being communicated about the client.

Malcolm felt very touched by the humanity of it all, of the sense of this little girl finding a voice, perhaps after so many years of silence, and of being heard. He wanted to check out how it had affected Laura and also to support her in being welcoming to this part of Jennifer.

'Very touching, very moving. Maybe you were the first person to really listen to that little girl.'

'I had that wonder. It felt so important to listen and not ask too many questions. I felt like I needed to make a relationship with this part of Jennifer. I really had to talk to her as I might do to a child. I mean, she was a child. There was not a sense of the adult Jennifer in the room.' Laura could feel her own eyes watering as she took herself back to the encounter. 'You know, I wonder why I didn't think of giving her a hug? I guess it was too soon. I mean, I know Jennifer, and I would not have a problem with hugging her in her adult state, but you know it never crossed my mind to reach out to Jennifer as the 7-year-old. I guess it would not have been appropriate, but thinking back now I have this real sense of her needing a hug, somehow, of some kind of reassurance that all will be OK.'

'You look surprised with yourself.'

'I am, and I feel that to have thought about and decided it was inappropriate to offer a hug would be one thing, but to simply not think about it at all is something else. I am feeling very affected as I sit here now, but somehow I wasn't feeling so affected at the time.'

'Any reflections on that?'

'I rather think I was getting caught up in the head and heart, or rather in the thoughts and feelings split that Jennifer mentioned afterwards, when she talked about knowing and feeling in relation to her changed view of her childhood. She was very shaken and upset when she began to realise that her view of her childhood as being happy may not be true. She talked of realising in her head that this was so, but was struggling to feel it. I think I got stuck in my head somehow, somewhere, with Jennifer as a little girl. But then, I do remember feeling I was relating to her as I would a child. I remember noticing that in myself.'

'Stuck in your head.'

'I don't think I was as in touch with feelings as I thought I was, looking back. And yet, thinking about it, I'm not sure how much feeling Jennifer as a child was expressing in that encounter. Let me think back for a moment.' Laura took herself back. 'She was afraid, she had a secret but couldn't, no, mustn't tell me because it would get her into trouble. She said her age and that she didn't have anyone to really talk to. It all sounded very matter of fact. And then she brightened and talked about her dolls. Did I miss something? Did I hold back? Was I in a place in myself that was going to be helpful for her? I'm wondering now.'

'Lots of questions . . . .'

'Yes, I really am wondering if I could have or should have been different. But maybe it was how it has to be for that first encounter. She may find it hard to trust people. One thing that does strike me is a sense of how she controlled what she said and what we talked about. Yes, now that I think back to it that feels very clear. But that is surely understandable. This is a very frightened part of her that has things she really wants to talk about, but wasn't able to. And she's carrying a secret.' Laura shivered. 'I do need to gain her trust and maybe I must trust how it is developing. I don't feel I did anything out of place. We have only just met.' Laura thought for a moment. 'You know, if Jennifer was aware of what was said during the encounter with her 7-year-old sense of self, I wonder if the 7-year-old is aware of the conversations Jennifer and I have had when she has been very much her adult self?'

'You wonder who knows what?'

'Something like that. But anyway, I know I need to be attentive to Jennifer the adult who is having to come to terms with her past, and Jennifer the little girl who I hope will feel able to come back again and talk some more. The more I think about it, the more it feels OK, and it is going to take time. And the hug concern does not feel such an issue anymore. But it does all leave Jennifer rather vulnerable, I think, and so she may call.'

Malcolm nodded. There was something nagging away at him, and he couldn't put it aside. Somehow when Laura had spoken about those dolls, it had seemed rather abrupt. Why had she mentioned the dolls? What did they mean?

'There's something troubling me, maybe more nagging at me, and it won't go away. You mentioned the three dolls, and somehow that seemed to get left hanging. Was that how it was, are we mirroring what Jennifer told you, or is there more to it? I'm just struck by the wonder of why she introduced the dolls.'

Malcolm has used his own experiencing to draw attention to an aspect of what Laura has been describing that he feels troubled by, though he does not know what it is. But he is open and sensitive enough to his own experience to be able to sense the presence of this nagging question. Much that is valuable in supervision can emerge from this kind of processing. The supervisor is reliant on what the supervisee tells him, and often it is only his own internal experiencing that can be used to register when something does not feel right, or is missing, or just doesn't quite add up.

The dolls. Laura thought back. 'Oh yes, I didn't mention it. She said Annabelle was her favourite, yes, her favourite because she was like her and needed to be cared for. How could I have not mentioned that? Oh and she liked dressing her up.'

'You forgot it?'

'Completely. Is that parallel-processing or my stuff? Why didn't I recall it?' Laura thought about it and she had no answer. 'It isn't that I didn't hear it, but after she had said it that part of her had gone.'

'So, my guess is that she was trying to tell you something, and the dolls were maybe a kind of metaphor, or more than a metaphor, for her own experience, perhaps? I'm being tentative here, I don't really want to try to interpret it, but she was I am sure trying to tell you something. The question is, did she feel heard?'

Laura looked and felt uncertain. 'I don't know. Maybe I missed it.' She thought back. 'No, I responded, and it was after my response, yes, immediately after my response, that she faded out.'

'Can you remember what you said?'

'Something like, "Annabelle is rather like you; she needs to be cared for, and you like dressing her up." '

'So it may be that she didn't feel heard and retreated, though it sounds like you did empathise with her quite accurately. So maybe she did feel heard and felt she had said enough at that time. Or maybe some other part of her thought she had said too much and stepped in and blocked her from saying more.'

'I need to think about why I forgot it here, though. It's important. She's telling me she needs to be cared for and I don't know that I really responded directly enough to that. I need to think about that. I wonder if I was reacting out of my own stuff? Silly question, of course I was, what else can I react out of other than myself?' Laura thought back to her own childhood. 'I had a reasonable childhood, a mixture of good and not so good. Did I feel cared for? Sometimes, but not always.'

'You may not necessarily be responding out of your own stuff from the past, of course.'

She smiled to herself. 'You know me too well, thank goodness. I need caring for too. Thinking about how much Jennifer needs Ian to care for her at the moment, and how much she doesn't want to think about the possibility of him not caring, brings me to a need for a little more caring in my own life. Every now and then I feel an urge to be back in a relationship, you know, although most of the time I feel good doing my own thing. I know what it is that may be happening. It's my own sensitivity towards my own feelings about being cared for that stopped me fully appreciating the power of what Jennifer was saying. I need to be more aware of that.' Laura stopped and thought. 'Yes, that was really helpful. My need to feel more cared for in my own life.'

When a supervisee appears to miss something when a client is discussing childhood issues it is easy to assume that the reason is something to do with the supervisee's childhood. As in this case, it may be something much more in the present and it is good practice that Malcolm is open to this and broadens Laura's focus out to include a consideration of what is more in Laura's present.

Laura continued, feeling she had gained the insight she needed and aware that time was passing by: 'Is there anything more you feel you need to know, as I don't feel I have much more to say, and there are some other issues with a couple of my other clients I want to mention.'

Malcolm gave himself a moment to check out his own thoughts and feelings about what Laura had been telling him. He felt he had an appreciation of the situation. He thought Laura was doing what needed to be done and that time would tell if memories were going to emerge either through what the 7-year-old Jennifer says or through other experiences when Jennifer was in her adult sense of self.

'No, I think that is OK. I think Jennifer has come a long way in the last few sessions and you have been there for her and with her during some difficult experiences. I'm sure you also need your break as well, and give yourself time to really experience yourself in your own world. We spend so much time exposed to our clients' inner worlds, we really do need time to be in our own as well! So, I shall be ready to listen if she calls and we'll see what emerges. Like you, I will want to trust the pace of her own process.'

Malcolm ended by asking Laura when she would be back and agreed to call her to let her know whether Jennifer had called or not. He said that if she called he would agree with her what he would pass on or whether he would leave it for her to tell Laura herself.

Telephone conversation

Jennifer had been back from her holiday for a week. She had enjoyed her time away but had still felt disturbed. The restless nights and the urge to drink in the evenings remained present, and she had begun to find herself losing interest in sex with her partner. He had been quite understanding, and she was relieved that it had not caused problems, but it wasn't making life easy, particularly as they had previously discussed and agreed to start a family.

She had been looking at Malcolm's phone number for a couple of days now, trying to decide whether or not to call. To begin with she had found it easy to decide not to, thinking that she would be troubling him and that she could wait for Laura to return. But she had had a particularly difficult night last night, three times she had woken up in a panic, sweating profusely, her heart pounding, and she had really struggled to calm down. She had briefly wondered if she was going mad, and she felt unable to say much to Ian. She couldn't really explain why, she just felt it was difficult somehow. She was again looking at the phone number. It was early evening. She had not had a drink but knew she was feeling sorely tempted. Ian wasn't home yet, and wasn't due back for a while. She felt wretched. She didn't know what to do. Two more weeks until she saw Laura seemed an age away.

She closed her eyes and took a deep breath, seeking to steady herself. She felt very shaky inside. Laura had told her that Malcolm was aware of the situation and that he was happy for her to call if need be. And she had said that he took calls around this time each day. It's no good, she thought to herself, I have to phone. I cannot go on like this. I have to talk to someone. I have to . . . . She wasn't sure what she needed, although there was a feeling of wanting some kind of reassurance.

She picked up the receiver and punched in the numbers on the slip of paper. She heard the pulses and the phone began to ring. She could feel her heart pounding as she waited for the receiver to be picked up.

'Hello, Malcolm here.'

'Oh, er, hello, um, my name's, um, Jennifer. Laura mentioned me to you? She said I might phone?'

'Yes, yes she did. Hello Jennifer. How can I help?'

'Have you time right now for me to talk?' Jennifer could feel so much tension within her as she asked this question, praying that he would say yes.

'Yes, I have. What's troubling you, Jennifer?' Malcolm could hear the trembling and anxiety in Jennifer's voice.

'Oh I feel awful.' Jennifer let out a long breath, swallowed and breathed in deeply.
    'Since I've been back from holiday, about a week now, I don't know, things

seem to be getting worse. I had a terrible night last night. My sleeping is really bad. I wake up with my heart thumping, feeling terrible. I feel I'm going mad. I just need to talk to someone, and, well, I would normally talk to Laura but she's away. So, oh God, am I making any sense? I feel at the end of my tether.'

'Yes, you are making sense but you feel it is driving you mad, at the end of your tether.'

'Yes.' Silence. 'Yes, I feel so wound up with it all, and I don't know what to do or what is happening.'

'Mmmm. Sounds desperate, I really hear the desperation in your voice, Jennifer.' Malcolm was aware that it might well turn into a telephone counselling session and he wanted to be sure that this was what Jennifer wanted. He didn't want to encourage this by his empathic responding unless he was sure that this was what she was seeking. 'And I guess I want to check out what you want from me now, whether you are looking for a telephone counselling session or if you feel you need to unload.'

'I don't know, I just feel I need to talk to someone who will understand or at least help me make sense of it all, even just a part of it. How long can you give me?'

Malcolm looked at the clock. He could offer Jennifer 20 minutes as he knew he would need some time for himself to process the conversation with Jennifer before his next session.

'Twenty minutes. Will that be OK?'

'Yes. I may not need that long, but I need to talk. Thank you.' Jennifer paused for a moment before continuing. Somehow she already felt a little easier, although she wasn't at all sure exactly why.

'So, I was hearing the desperation in your voice.'

'Yes, well, I feel I'm bottling things up and it's putting me under pressure. Let me tell you what has been happening and maybe that will help. Is that OK?'

'OK by me, please talk about whatever you feel you need to.' Malcolm genuinely meant this as he said it. He didn't know what Jennifer needed to talk about and felt sure that she would know, even though she might take a while to get to it.

Jennifer noted how genuine that had sounded. 'Well, the holiday – I found myself drinking each evening, and drinking more than I usually do, not just a bottle of wine with the meal, but there would be apéritifs and we would often spend time in the bar in the evenings. I got a bit out of order a few times, I got argumentative with Ian, my partner, and, well, I can't remember it all that clearly. I drank far too much the last night and apparently made something of a scene, and, oh I don't know, ended up having a blazing row with Ian. I can't really remember what happened but the flight back, well, we didn't speak very much. I know I had a few more drinks, and since we've been back I've really struggled. And I've really had to fight against the urge to drink more. You know I had a drink problem in the past?'

'Yes, Laura had mentioned that.'

'OK, well, I'm afraid that it will get out of control again, and mess up my relationship, and all at a time when we had begun to seriously talk about starting a family.' With this Malcolm could hear the sound of sobbing down the phone.

'I really hear that fear, Jennifer, so much that you don't want to mess up . . . .'

He deliberately left his response open, waiting to hear what Jennifer would choose to focus on.

'I've been so happy and now I feel so wretched.' The sobs became more frequent and Jennifer could feel the tears running down her face. 'I need to get a tissue. Just a minute.'

Malcolm waited. It seemed like an age. Thoughts passed through his mind. Was she OK? Had she switched into a dissociated silence? Might she open herself to feelings that she could not control? Would she be on her own the rest of the evening and how would she cope? He closed his eyes and refocused himself, recognising that his thinking was running away with itself. Now, let's be calm about this, he said to himself. I need to be here to listen to what Jennifer wants to say, and if I still feel concerned I can ask some of these questions later if they persist and feel relevant. He waited, and heard the phone being picked up.

He heard Jennifer breathing out heavily. 'I think I needed that, needed to release some of those tears. I am so afraid of losing it.'

'So afraid of losing what you have?'

'Yes. I need to make sense of what is happening. But I can't, I just know that something doesn't feel right within me. The waking up, the dreams. I don't usually dream, or at least, I don't seem to remember them very clearly. But now, well, now I am getting a sense of what some of them are about, and they always seem to involve me feeling trapped, unable to get away from something, or someone. I wake up sometimes with what feels like a huge pressure on my chest, but I guess that's my heart pounding.'

'So you can't relax but you are having dreams that you are kind of remembering a little about, and they involve feeling trapped, unable to get away, feeling of pressure on your body.'

Malcolm was very mindful of the discussions he had had with Laura as to what might be behind what Jennifer was experiencing, but he knew he was there to listen and allow Jennifer to explore and make her own sense of her experience. His sense, though, was that experiences were coming to the surface through the dreaming process and the sense that she had had of pressure on her chest made him think that further, clearer imagery could be very close. He wondered when Laura was next seeing Jennifer as he could feel his own concern as to whether she might experience some flashbacks before then and need support. But he also didn't want to alarm Jennifer or put ideas into her head as to anything that might be behind her experiences. He knew that when he had said 'pressure on your body', he may have overstepped the mark. She had said 'pressure on my chest'. His response had in a way extended what was being described and might push Jennifer towards something she was not yet ready to recognise, this all assuming that some form of sexual abuse lay behind Jennifer's current difficulties. He realised that he needed to explore this in his own supervision.

There was no response from Jennifer. Malcolm could feel the silence incredibly acutely. He remembered how Laura had described the way that Jennifer could flip back into that child-like self, and had passed out completely on one occasion. 'Jennifer,' he said softly, 'I am still here if there is something more that you want to say.'

The silence continued. Jennifer was conscious, but she was miles away from the phone conversation, well actually years away, in her past. She did hear Malcolm's voice, but it had seemed very distant. She wasn't really remembering anything specific, but it was as though she was held in suspension, not really thinking or feeling, just sitting. She felt small, very small. She became aware that she was rocking gently backwards and forwards, backwards and forwards, again and again and again. This wasn't just a memory, she was aware that this was what she was doing as she sat there holding the phone. She could hear Malcolm's voice, this time it sounded quite urgent. 'Jennifer, are you OK, can you let me know if you can hear me?'

'Yes, yes, I can. Sorry. I . . . I'm not sure what happened. I just . . . I don't know. I heard your voice just now, you sounded really concerned and I remember hearing you say you were there if there was something else I wanted to say.'

'How are you now, Jennifer?'

'Not sure. Numb. I feel quite . . . numb, it's the only word that comes to mind. I somehow feel much calmer. I don't understand.'

'Numb, as though what you had been feeling has somehow been, well, kind of taken away?'

'Yes, like it feels distant. But that can't be. I mean, I . . . I do feel different but I don't feel right. I don't feel me. It's like I feel kind of drugged somehow. As though, as though part of me is missing but I know it isn't really?'

'Part of you is missing but it isn't really.' Malcolm responded directly to the last part of what Jennifer had said.

'Yes. What were we talking about before this happened?'

Malcolm felt his jaw tighten. He knew it had been that comment about pressure on her body. He didn't want to lead her, but then saying those words had clearly had a profound effect on Jennifer, and he had to trust the process here. No sense in being anything other than authentic.

'You were talking about how you felt when you woke up after the disturbing dreams you had been having. I said something like you are remembering the dreams involve feeling trapped, unable to get away, feeling of pressure on your body.'

'Yes, not feeling able to breathe, I get that.' Jennifer was aware of somehow feeling distant from her dreams though, distant from those feelings. She shook her head and noticed that time had passed, almost 15 minutes since she had started the call. 'I think I flipped back into that place in myself that I have been in with Laura. It all feels so weird and yet somehow I feel easier having just had that experience and talking to you. I think that it had all built up and I needed to let the pressure out. I really appreciate you listening and letting me talk and be silent.'

Sometimes people just need a little time to release thoughts and feelings, and to experience someone else listening and giving them quality attention. When a sense of feeling overwhelmed arises it can leave people with all kinds of self-doubts, and experiences can grow out of proportion, fuelled by mounting anxiety. The reassurance of someone listening and taking them seriously can be extremely helpful and can help the person to regain control. This was appropriate in this case as the aim was to offer support for Jennifer during Laura's absence, to help her through anything difficult that might arise.

'That's OK. So you feel a little easier now, less bottled up?'

'Yes, yes. I think my head was spinning with it all and I couldn't get it out. And that strange silence seems to have somehow calmed me down too.'

Malcolm was aware that time was passing. 'I'm glad things feel a little easier for you. I am also aware that we only have a few more minutes.'

'OK, look, I feel a lot better having talked to you, Malcolm, and I really hope you don't mind me calling, I really am grateful. I know that the time is nearly up.'

'I'm glad you called and that things have eased. Sometimes it is better to take the pressure off a little and no doubt when Laura returns you can explore it more deeply.'

'Yes.' Jennifer paused. 'I want to pay you for your time, is that OK?'

Malcolm gave Jennifer his hourly rate and she agreed to send him a cheque in the post. They also agreed that she could phone again if she needed to, with the same financial arrangement, and that if things felt too much then maybe they could arrange a definite time for a telephone counselling contact. Jennifer was grateful for this idea but felt that maybe she would wait to see how things went and she hoped she could wait to see Laura. She agreed that she would let Laura know that she had spoken to Malcolm but also agreed that he could talk about the telephone contact with Laura when he next saw her. She felt reassured in herself knowing that she could call Malcolm if she needed to. It also kind of felt good that he was supervising Laura as well.

The phone call ended and Malcolm slowly put down the receiver. That had been an intense session, he was aware that his level of concentration had been really intense. He found this generally when counselling over the phone, trying to pick up on the tone of voice and to be in relationship with a client when the only active sense that could be used was hearing. And, of course, this was his first direct contact with Jennifer. He needed a glass of water and time to clear his head. He jotted down his thoughts and reflections and began to get himself ready for his next face-to-face client.

Points for discussion

- Evaluate your own use of empathy in terms of whether your tone of voice, or emphasis on words, has a directing effect on clients.

- How does a counsellor's own experience of childhood make it difficult for them to genuinely hear what the client may convey about their's, particularly when, as with Jennifer, she is confronted with an awareness that it was not as she had believed it to be?
- Had you been the client, would you have felt Laura's responses to have been what you wanted/needed to hear?
- Do you think more might have been said or explored with the client with regard to her having Malcolm's number. If so, what?
- What are your thoughts and reactions concerning Malcolm's use of his own sensed feelings and thoughts within the supervision session?
- What were your reactions to the telephone conversation?
- What would have been your concerns if the silence had continued longer and what responses would you have made?

CHAPTER 5

Counselling session 37

Jennifer arrived a couple of minutes early and sat outside in her car, collecting her thoughts and preparing herself for the session. The conversation with Malcolm had certainly helped although she could not explain why. At least it had for a few days, but the dreams had come back at her again, she had continued to wake up feeling very disturbed and had not managed to change her evening drinking pattern. She had also had two particularly disturbing dreams in which she had seen her father's face very clearly, and had felt tremendous fear. She wasn't sure what that was about and she wanted to talk about them this evening.

Time had passed, and she got out of the car, went up to the door and rang the bell. Laura let her in. She noticed she seemed to have quite a tan. 'You look like you had a good holiday!'

Laura smiled. She had, but didn't want to get side-tracked into small talk about her holiday. 'Yes, thanks.' She led the way into the counselling room. They sat down.

'I spoke to Malcolm on one occasion, after I got back, and it was helpful, although I don't feel anything has really changed. Still feeling disturbed, still sleeping badly, dreaming weird dreams.'

'So, nothing has really changed since I last saw you?'

'Well, I was telling Malcolm about my holiday, how I drank a bit too much and it led to arguments with Ian. I didn't mention it to Malcolm but I began to have trouble feeling interested in sex, couldn't feel aroused.'

'Seems to me like a lot has been going on for you. The holiday caused tensions between you and Ian with the drinking and losing interest in sex.'

'Yes. Still not really interested in sex. I just feel I go cold at the thought of it, and that's not like me. I just can't get into the mood at all. I love Ian, I really do, and I do like feeling close to him, but when it comes to arousal and to inter-course, I just can't. I have noticed though that I am often thinking about this when I drink. I hadn't been doing that before, but I somehow find myself get-ting really tense in the evenings when I think about going to bed at night, and I do begin to think that drinking has become a way of dealing with this.'

'Drinking reduces some of the tensions that you are feeling around sex but you don't want to be drinking like this.' Laura could see the sadness in Jennifer's eyes. 'I see so much sadness in your eyes, Jennifer, so much sadness.'

Empathic responding to what is being communicated by facial expression and body language can be a powerful intervention. The mind can censor what is communicated, but the body can be much more transparent.

Jennifer could feel the sadness rising in her as she heard Laura speak. Yes, she was feeling so sad, and the tears began to flow from her eyes. 'I don't understand what is happening to me, Laura, I really don't. And I have been having awful, troubling dreams. I've even started having them about my father and I don't understand that, I really don't.'

'Dreams of your father?' Laura responded in a way to encourage further clarification.

'I've had dreams in which I have seen his face, his face as he was, oh, 20 or 25 years or so ago, when he didn't have a beard like he does now.' Jennifer stopped for a moment, and bit her lower lip. 'I see his face, it's close to mine, and I feel frightened. I feel very frightened.'

'Very frightened as you look at his clean-shaven face.' Laura sought to try to hold Jennifer on the image she had described, communicating back what she had heard her describe.

Jennifer nodded and lowered her head. She began to rock to and fro. Laura could see Jennifer seemingly getting smaller as she sat in the chair. She's shifting back into her past again, Laura thought, and immediately sought to sharpen her concentration and openness to what was present in the relationship and in herself. The rocking continued and a couple of minutes passed.

Laura was aware of the previous session when Jennifer had spoken as a child. She wondered if she might be able to facilitate this part of Jennifer to communicate again. Laura spoke softly and simply. 'I'd like to hear you if you have something you want to tell me.' She waited.

'Can't tell you. Mustn't tell you. Be a bad girl if I tell you.'

'Can't tell me, mustn't tell me. You feel you'll be a bad girl if you do.'

Laura does not simply reflect back the last sentence, not wishing to re-enforce the idea that Jennifer *is* a bad girl, rather that this was what she is *feeling* about herself.

'Yes.' Jennifer looked up and rolled her head to one side. 'Don't listen to her. She doesn't know what she's talking about.'

'Who am I talking to?' Laura knew that the voice she was hearing was not the same one as she had heard before.

'We talked last time.'

'Yes, I remember, you had something you couldn't tell me as well?'

'Yes, well I don't any more.'

'Don't any more?'

'No.' The room went silent again. 'Can we play a game?'

'What game would you like to play?'

'Best friends.' The voice had changed again, younger, much younger.

'I don't know that one. How do you play it?'

'You touch me.'

'I touch you?'

'Yes.'

Laura thought for a moment. She was not sure how much Jennifer as an adult was aware of this conversation but she felt intuitively that she had to continue. Part of Jennifer was emerging and she needed to listen to what it wanted to tell her.

'Is that the game?'

'Yes.'

'Who taught you the game of best friends, Jennifer?'

'Daddy did. We play it when he comes home from work.'

'You and daddy play best friends when he comes home from work?'

'Yes.'

Laura noted that Jennifer was silent and she felt she wanted to maintain the dialogue with the part of Jennifer that had emerged, sensing that the other part might cut in and block what was being said. She knew the question that she had to ask, 'How do you play this game? How do you touch?'

'Daddy lets me touch him, touch him here below his tummy. He calls it his worm and he says it's friendly and wants to be my friend too.'

Laura could feel the hairs on the back of her neck standing on end and the goose bumps breaking out on her back and neck. Oh shit, oh shit, she hadn't expected that, quite so bluntly. What next?

'He says the worm wants to be your friend too?'

'Yes, but sometimes it's not friendly, sometimes it hurts me, bites me, hurts me.'

Laura fought back the temptation to close her eyes. She could feel them moistening as she listened to the words being spoken from somewhere deep within Jennifer, some part of her that had been hidden back in the past. She kept her eyes open, looking at Jennifer and allowing herself to feel the surge of compassion that arose within her.

'Not so friendly, hurts you, bites you.' Laura deliberately kept her words simple. The voice she was hearing sounded so much younger than the other one that had spoken before and in the last session.

'Yes, hurts me, bites me. Don't like it.'

Laura could feel herself going cold. She wanted to ask how old this part of Jennifer was but she also wanted to help her say more if she could, if she wanted to. She knew she had to trust Jennifer's process. What was being said was being said at this time for a reason. She had to trust that Jennifer was ready to face up to what was being said, to distant experiences that had been dissociated and which had remained locked up within herself.

'You don't like it hurting and biting you.'

'No.' A tear ran down her right cheek, her eyes became quite watery. 'But he says I'm a good girl, but it hurts.'

'Can you tell me where it hurts you and bites you?' As soon as she said it Laura bit her lip, feeling she had pushed Jennifer into a maybe difficult disclosure.

> Working at depth with dissociated parts within the client requires great sensitivity and an ability to stay very close to the client in order to maintain contact. The part of Jennifer that is speaking is obviously vulnerable and is going to easily shy away, it has only just found its voice and is likely to need an encouraging and warmly accepting relationship to continue. Anything that threatens it, or draws other parts out that might silence the part that is speaking is unhelpful. Laura has strayed from this and is now at risk of losing contact with the part that is speaking.

Jennifer's face changed and it became almost angelic. 'Can't tell you, mustn't tell you.'

'You can't tell me, mustn't tell me where daddy's worm hurt you and bit you.' Laura could feel herself struggling to say the words, they stuck in her throat as she spoke them. They felt like glass cutting into her and yet she tried to say them softly and gently, not wishing to push Jennifer to say more than she felt able to at this time.

Jennifer shook her head, and began to cry.

'Always crying.' The voice had changed back to the older little girl. 'I don't like her.'

'Don't like her?'

'No. And she's told you, hasn't she? She's told you.' Fear had spread across Jennifer's face.

'Yes, she has told me.'

'Hmm. Well, he did it to me too. But I don't cry.'

'Did it to you too, but you don't cry.'

'No. I don't cry, I'm braver than she is.'

'You don't cry and you are braver.' Laura wanted to reach out to this part of Jennifer that had clearly found a way of surviving which involved not crying and perhaps not feeling either. She wondered momentarily at how these aspects of Jennifer had remained invisible, particularly during the counselling over the previous months.

'Yes. But I've got to go now. We've got to go now.'

'OK, you both have to go now. Thank you for talking to me. I really hope we can talk again.' Laura wondered at what she had just said. In one sense it felt surreal, but at the same time it all felt extremely real.

Silence again, but this was different. This was not the silence she had experienced before. Jennifer no longer looked or felt small. This was Jennifer back as the adult. She could see the look of absolute horror on her face. Jennifer burst into tears. She sobbed, she wailed, she repeated the words again and again, 'Oh no, not me, not me.' Laura could not just sit and observe the distress that was pouring out of Jennifer. She got up and knelt down next to her, taking her in her arms. The tears continued to flow and the distress pulled at Laura's heart. 'No, no, not me, not me.' The words hung in the room each time, they seemed to burn into the pit of Laura's stomach, like red hot needles. Laura acknowledged her own feelings yet knew that they were nothing to what Jennifer was experiencing.

Minutes passed, the tears continued to flow, Laura held Jennifer as her body shook with the pain of the sudden insight that had burst upon her. She felt as if her whole being was tearing apart, like molten lava was flowing through her veins. She burned. She hurt. No thoughts, just overwhelming feelings all over her body.

Laura could feel the tears in her own eyes as she knelt next to Jennifer. She was very conscious of a sense of womanly solidarity. It was as though they were somehow sharing a pain that was part of a greater pain in the world. It felt overwhelming but she knew she had to hold this and be ready for Jennifer and able to listen to whatever else she needed to say. She could feel Jennifer clinging to her as she sobbed, feel the tension in her grip. She sought to convey her empathy for Jennifer by endeavouring to match her grip with her own. Eventually she felt Jennifer's grip relax a little and she relaxed hers too.

> Empathic sensitivity to the experiencing of the client can be effectively communicated through physical contact, and where sensitively offered in a context where physical contact has caused pain, can be powerfully reassuring for the client. Not only do the mind and the heart need to be heard, so too does the body.

'Oh God.' Jennifer said nothing more as she loosened her grip further. She looked into Laura's eyes and shook her head. 'I can't believe it but I know it.' She was aware that she had started to go numb. 'I – I don't know what to do.' The hesitancy was clear in her voice. 'I feel like I have woken up to a terrible, terrible nightmare. I can't believe it, but I heard myself ... I heard myself.' Jennifer closed her eyes, she could feel the emotion rising again and the tears streamed back out of her eyes. She leaned over and put her head on Laura's shoulder and continued to cry, the tide of emotion bursting upon her. 'Thank God you're here, Laura, thank God you're here.'

Laura responded by gently rubbing Jennifer's back. She didn't need to say anything. She knew she was very present and that Jennifer was aware of this.

> Empathy can be conveyed in many ways, and in this situation it is being conveyed through physical contact. It does, however, raise issues where the counsellor is of the gender that is the sexual preference of the client, or vice versa.

> If Jennifer's counsellor was a heterosexual male, could he feel inhibited to openly offer physical contact to support Jennifer in her anguish? And how might Jennifer react and interpret such an intervention? Often the decision to initiate physical contact from the counsellor flows out of a sense of 'rightness' in the moment that is a product of the presence of therapeutic relationship and empathic rapport.
>
> Where there is hesitancy or uncertainty it is perhaps more appropriate to ask the client if they need to be physically held.

Jennifer felt supported by Laura's presence. Whilst she felt suddenly very lonely she also felt a strong connection to Laura. It gave her strength. She took a deep breath and opened her eyes again. She let go of Laura and reached over for a tissue, drying her eyes and blowing her nose. 'I'm OK now.'

Laura took that as her cue to return to her seat but she felt she wanted to check this first. 'OK for me to go back to my seat?'

'Yes.' Jennifer nodded her head as she spoke, still unable to really take it all in. She sat, staring at the wall. 'I feel so much and I don't know what to feel. Does that make sense?'

Laura felt herself nodding. 'Too much to know what to feel.' She resisted answering the question, choosing to allow it to remain unanswered and therefore more likely that Jennifer might find her own response without it being coloured by Laura's reaction.

'I don't know what to feel. I feel so much and yet I feel numb at the same time. I . . . .' Jennifer shook her head again. 'I . . .' and let out a deep breath, blowing the air out of her mouth and drawing her lips together as she breathed back in through her nose, tightening them into a grimace.

'Seems like there is nothing to say . . . and so much to say.' Laura sought to empathise with Jennifer's struggle to find words at a time and in a place when perhaps there were no words, not yet anyway, for what must be so present for her. No doubt other feelings such as anger would emerge in time, but Jennifer was not there yet. She had been hit by a hurricane of feelings and was in emotional shock. She needed time to be, and for a companion to be with her.

'I don't know what to do, Laura, I just don't know what to do.' She continued to sit in silence staring ahead of her. She felt so strange. There were no real thoughts as such, more of an emptiness, yet her emotions also felt like they had been hit by a truck. She did feel very weak, though, a weakness that seemed to sit throughout her body. Her arms felt heavy and slightly tingly, like a kind of itch in her veins. Her legs, well she knew they were there but they felt like a dead weight. They didn't feel like they were her legs somehow. Her breathing was very shallow. 'I feel like I'm . . . like I'm paralysed by it all. I feel like I could just sit here forever.' Jennifer closed here eyes again and began to shake her head.

Laura said nothing, allowing Jennifer to remain undisturbed in her paralysed state. This was probably exactly what her body needed at this time. No stimulation but rather time to recover from the emotional onslaught that had occurred. She felt she was being empathic to Jennifer's unexpressed organismic need. She continued to sit quietly, ensuring that she maintained heightened attention on Jennifer.

Jennifer moved her head and looked at Laura again. Again she shook her head. She could not believe what was happening, had happened. She could feel the numbness in her face as she sat, and her eyes felt so heavy. She took in another deep breath and let it go, feeling her chest relax as she did so. She became aware of the tightness in her back, just below the shoulder blades and she moved her shoulders to try to free it off, and stretched to try and unlock the constriction. It helped a little. She rolled her neck slightly, aware also of the tension that was there.

She looked across at Laura again and into her deep blue eyes. They seemed to be so full of compassion and caring. Sometimes her eyes had felt quite searching but not now. She could see her own hurt mirrored in them, and that felt so reassuring too.

'It really happened, didn't it? I was sexually abused by my father.'

'Yes, it really happened, he sexually abused you.'

'I can't believe it but I do believe it. I want to deny it, but I heard myself speaking.' Jennifer shook her head.

Jennifer has regained her awareness of her being sexually abused through experiencing the words from dissociated parts of herself. Often the remembering may come through dreams and flashbacks, with the survivor at times doubting the reality of what has emerged into their awareness. Bass and Davis (1988, p. 347) stress the importance of the counsellor continuing to believe that their client was sexually abused throughout the counselling process, even if the client doubts it themself. 'Doubting,' they say, 'is part of the process of coming to terms with abuse.'

After a silence Jennifer spoke again. 'Thanks.'

Laura smiled, tight-lipped, she could feel her compassion for Jennifer. 'That's OK. You have had an horrendous realisation, I just feel so much for you and want to help you through it.'

Jennifer felt her eyes watering again. She could feel the caring. She didn't think she had ever felt this depth of caring, ever. She could feel the tears trickling down her cheeks, she closed her eyes again and gritted her teeth. Another deep breath.

'What now?' Jennifer asked the question, aware that time was passing by. The session was close to ending but she still felt so heavy and tired.

'Take your time, get up when you are ready. You look as though you are glued in the chair.'

A slight smile appeared on Jennifer's face. 'Yes, that's how I feel. And I've got to get home. I'm really not sure if I am together enough to do that.'

'Not sure if you can handle the drive?'

'No, I really feel that I need to call Ian and ask him to come and pick me up. Would it be OK to leave the car outside overnight?'

Laura had no problem with that and said as much. She asked if Jennifer wanted to use her phone but she said she had her mobile, then Laura asked if she wanted privacy to make the call. Jennifer said that she would appreciate that. 'Do you fancy a cup of tea while you are waiting?'

'Yes, thanks, I'd really appreciate that.'

It can arise that a client does not feel that they are in a fit state to make their way home. In this case, Jennifer has recognised this for herself and has made arrangements for her partner to come and pick her up. It could have been that she might have needed to call a taxi. Either way, the effect is that the client remains beyond the counselling session and the question then arises as to how this should be handled. It could be that another client is due and it is impractical for the client to stay in the room. Is there another room she can wait in, or might she have to wait in the car? The latter is an option, however, given the nature of the session this would seem inappropriate. Laura has taken the decision to be with her until Ian arrives. From a person-centred perspective this is surely a human response, a warm acceptance of Jennifer and an authentic empathic appreciation of the situation as far as Jennifer is concerned. What, though, do you talk about when the session has ended without getting back into therapy again?

Laura left the room. When she returned with the tea, Jennifer was sitting quietly looking out of the window. She didn't turn as Laura came in but spoke softly. 'You know, everything has changed now, hasn't it? I mean, I can never be the same person. I don't feel the same person.'

'Everything has changed?' Laura responded with an empathic question and awaited Jennifer's response.

'Well, I mean, I guess I . . . .' Jennifer was aware she was at a loss for words. She just knew she felt different and somehow in that moment of revelation she had changed forever. 'I can't get it into words.' She turned and tightened her lips as she looked at Laura and took the mug of tea. 'Thanks.'

'Everything has changed but it is hard to define the change, and maybe that will all take time?' Laura added the second bit to try to help reassure Jennifer who seemed to be struggling to try to make sense of it as she sat there.

Laura has made the decision to engage with Jennifer, perhaps realising that in these few minutes before Ian arrives there may be time for her to begin to process what has occurred in the session and the effect it has had on her. She trusted her to know best how she wanted to use the time. This trusting of the client to know what their needs are in the present Laura knew to be a core feature of person-centred working.

'Yes, it will take time. And I guess I'm sitting here knowing that there are chunks of my childhood that I don't remember, you know, things about what happened to me as a child. I don't have the memories and I guess I really don't know whether or not I want them.' It's like being told there is something scary behind the door – a bit of me wants to know what it is, and the rest wants the door shut, not just shut, boarded up so what's in there can't get out. Yet somehow it has got out, hasn't it, and I can't really put it back.' She could feel a sudden rush of insight. 'That's why I drink, isn't it. Evenings. Shutting feelings out.' She shivered.

'I hear your mixed feelings about remembering. Part of you wants to board them up in a closet, another part wants to know what they are.' Laura didn't get a chance to finish what she was saying as Jennifer interrupted.

'I don't want to drink on this, I really don't, but I know I'm going to want to, and . . . .'

'You know you're going to want to drink on it but you don't want to.'

'Yes, but I mustn't. It's going to take time to come to terms with all of this.' She sipped at her tea. 'But I have to keep going, people do, don't they?'

'Yes, people do.' Laura spoke slowly as she responded. She added, wanting to try and validate and show some acceptance of whatever Jennifer chose to do, 'You will find your own way through it, I see you as a strong woman. I really mean that.'

Jennifer smiled. 'We shall see. Can I see you weekly for a while? I'd really appreciate that.'

'Yes, you can. And I can probably make it the same time and day. And if you need to call and talk, that's OK.]'

'Thanks, that feels good.' She took more sips from her tea. 'OK. I need time to reflect, talk with Ian, I need time to kind of recover. Yet I also know that there's going to be more, isn't there?'

Laura nodded. There wasn't any point in denying it. Jennifer was perfectly right. She knew she had to trust Jennifer to make the choices that were right for her. She wanted to come more and that maybe indicated that the part of her that wanted to work through it was dominating her decision making. But she was also aware that it might not remain that way.

The two of them sat in silence for a while. Laura wondered whether she had blurred the counselling boundaries, but took comfort in her belief that her action was flowing from her unconditional positive regard for Jennifer.

'Lot to think about,' Laura commented, 'and we'll take it at the pace that you want to go at.'

'I couldn't be rushed. Not enough energy.'

The doorbell rang. Ian had arrived. He looked worried. 'How is Jennifer?' he asked.

'I'll leave it for her to talk to you.' Laura was mindful of confidentiality. She did not know what Jennifer had said to Ian on the phone and she was grateful not to have said something like 'She's had quite a shock.' Maybe Jennifer hadn't said what had happened, she might have just said she had come over feeling unwell.

Jennifer appeared in the doorway, looking a bit wobbly and pale. 'Hi.'

'You look all in. Come on, let's get you home.'

They went out of the door together. 'Thanks, Laura, I'll see you next week.'

'OK. Look after yourself.'

'I will, and I've got Ian to look after me too.'

Laura closed the door as they reached the garden gate. She turned and walked back into the counselling room, sat down and just spent time being with what she was feeling. She felt absolutely wiped out, and realised just how much the session had taken out of her. She had to force herself to write up her brief notes of the session. She was glad that she had had something to eat before the session, she certainly didn't feel like cooking now. But the washing up was waiting for her. She looked at it, thought about it, and decided to leave it for a moment. She poured herself another cup of tea and went into the front room to see if there was something mindless on TV – there usually was – but even that didn't help her switch off. She tried some relaxing music but that didn't seem to make any impression either. She realised that she didn't need something to unwind, rather something to help her release. Finally she played the overture from Tannhauser – she knew the surging strings would have the effect she needed. It did. She cried and allowed her emotions to surge through her. Afterwards, she felt very quiet and still, and a lot better. She attended to the washing up.

Within this session has emerged the presence of more than one distinctive identity within Jennifer's self-structure. In the past this phenomenon might have been labelled as 'multiple personality disorder', however, from a person-centred perspective it could be seen more as being nearer dissociative identity disorder. Jennifer, in her childhood, has generated within herself at least two dissociative identities as a method of coping with and surviving the psychologically overwhelming nature of the experience of being sexually abused. What is important from the person-centred perspective is that whilst these identities have a distinctive nature, they are actually bound together within a single process. There is interaction between them, and now, through what has emerged within the session, this interaction has impacted on the conscious awareness of Jennifer as an adult.

The following morning Jennifer had returned to pick up the car, but Laura had already gone out. When Laura returned later that day she noticed the car had gone and on the front doormat was an envelope. Inside was a card from Jennifer:

Dear Laura,

Thanks for yesterday. I somehow had a good night's sleep last night, and didn't drink. Too tired. Just went to bed. Feeling better now, more energy. Going out for a walk in the countryside. See you next week. Thanks again for your support. I really appreciated it.

With gratitude, Jennifer.

Laura has sought to give Jennifer time to be with what she has been experiencing throughout the session. She provided a steady presence throughout the process in which the revelation that Jennifer had been a victim of sexual abuse in childhood emerged. Providing this steady, consistent presence will have been valued by Jennifer. Sitting there listening to the two aspects of her childhood talking, and hearing what was being said, would have been extremely shocking and traumatic. Jennifer is a woman who had completely repressed the memories of what happened. She still cannot recall events, all that she knows is her fear when waiting at the window, and the knowing that something occurred with her father and that it hurt her.

Laura offers telephone support if necessary, recognising the degree of fragility that Jennifer will be experiencing. This is a responsible course of action to take. It will feel like a long week for Jennifer before the next session.

Counselling session 38

It had gone 7.30pm and Laura was sitting waiting for Jennifer and was aware that she was experiencing anxiety. She had not heard from Jennifer at all since that card, the morning after the last session. Part of her wanted to believe that it was because she was coping, but she could not deny her anxiety that perhaps things had taken a turn for the worse, causing Jennifer to decide that she could not face another session, or that her drinking had increased and was possibly the cause of her not attending. The minutes passed as Laura waited. She couldn't put her concerns aside, they were too present. She thought of phoning Jennifer but she knew that the agreement they had was that if she did not attend, Laura would wait and call the next day.

She told herself that Jennifer was making the choice that she needed to make to deal with what she was feeling. She felt her lips tighten as she thought about that, and how lovely it sounded. But what about when you introduce a mood-altering chemical into that cocktail of experience? The kind of fragile place that Jennifer had entered into and the possibility of excess alcohol left her concerned for Jennifer's safety. Laura was mindful of something she had read recently about clients in 'fragile process'.

The idea is that clients who as children experienced 'empathic failure' went on to 'experience a "fragile" style of processing as adults .... Clients who have a fragile style of processing tend to experience core issues at very high or low levels of intensity. They tend to have difficulty starting and stopping experiences that are personally significant or emotionally connected' (Warner, 2000, p. 150).

It was getting on for a quarter to eight. Jennifer usually arrived promptly. Laura felt the temptation to get up and make a tea for herself, but she decided to continue to sit. She decided that maybe she should just sit and hold Jennifer gently in her thoughts.

She closed her eyes and visualised Jennifer sitting in front of her, and just sought to allow her feelings of warmth and caring to reach out to her. She was very gentle with this process, and could feel quite a profound quietness settling upon her as she sat there. She felt her anxiety ease somewhat. Somehow she found herself feeling a little more reassured that whatever was happening for Jennifer would be OK. It would probably be extremely distressing, but she had a faith that she would come through. Or was it simply her own hope that she desperately wanted to keep alive? She did not know. As she thought about it she felt her anxiety returning.

The phone rang and she nearly jumped out of her skin. She certainly felt as if she had left the chair, her heart suddenly pounding. She shook her head and got up, making her way to the phone in the hall.

'Hello, Laura speaking.'

'Hello Laura. It's Ian, Jennifer's partner, we met briefly last week.'

'Yes, hello. I was, er, due to see Jennifer this evening but she hasn't arrived.'

'No, she's here. I have just got home myself. She's been drinking and she's not going to make it to you. She really has had a bad week, though not every day, and not drinking every day. But the last couple of evenings she really has gone for it. She seems to want to drink to fall asleep. She's making it in to work but I'm not sure how well she's functioning. Do you want to have a word with her? She knows I'm phoning you. I think she feels so bad about not letting you know, and about what she is doing to herself at the moment.'

'Yes, I'll speak to her if that's what she wants.'

'Thanks.' Laura heard Ian talking to Jennifer, telling her that Laura was on the phone and would be happy to talk to her if she wanted to.

'I'm so sorry, I'm so sorry. I've let you down. I'm so sorry.' Jennifer's words were slurring a little and she sounded very distant. Laura realised that she was relieved to hear Jennifer and to know that she was OK even though she was drinking. She knew that she needed to let Jennifer know that she was there for her, that this was not going to stop the counselling continuing, and that she, Laura, didn't feel let down. But she hoped she could introduce these things as the conversation developed.

'I was feeling anxious for you, Jennifer, but it's good to hear your voice.'

'I'm struggling to cope, Laura, I'm struggling to cope. I've had a bad week, a bad week . . . .' Jennifer's voice trailed off.

'Do you want to tell me about it, Jennifer?'

Laura has made the decision to offer Jennifer the opportunity to talk if she wants to. She is unsure what Jennifer feels her needs are at this time, and what she hopes to gain from speaking to her. She does not want to try to

> impose anything on Jennifer, but to offer her space if she wants to use it. She knows that she needs to ensure that the therapeutic relationship can be preserved.

'I just lost the plot yesterday evening, and again tonight. I feel so wretched, so confused, so awful, so bloody awful. Ian's been great, he really has. I don't deserve him.' Laura could hear Jennifer beginning to cry.

'Hard to feel good about anything at the moment, Jennifer, but he's been there for you, and he's there for you now.'

'Yes, I know.' Laura could hear how Jennifer was struggling to speak through the tears. 'I've got to stop the drinking, Laura, I know why I'm drinking, it's just so hard.' The crying intensified. 'I just keep wondering about the past, about what happened and I just want to blot it all out, blot it out before I really know what it is. And I know I can't do that for the rest of my life. I've got to face it, but it's so hard, it's so, so hard.'

Laura could hear the desperation in Jennifer's voice. 'I really hear how desperately hard it is, Jennifer, and I want you to know that I really want to help you work this through.' Laura could feel her emotions rising as she spoke.

Jennifer could also hear the feelings behind the words although it was a little hazy. That bottle of wine she had consumed earlier on an empty stomach when she got home early from work was having more and more of an effect on her. She could feel herself drifting more and more. 'Look, I'm feeling bad and I'm going to have to go. Can I make an appointment for next week?'

'Sure, same time, same day.'

'OK. I'm really going to try, I really need to do this. My father's fucked me up and I don't want it any more. Fucked me up! Bloody says it all, doesn't it? Bastard. I don't fucking want it any more.' Jennifer could feel the anger in herself, a boiling rage that seemed to have overwhelmed her.

'Yeah, sounds powerful, you don't fucking want it any more.'

'No I don't.' Jennifer's voice had returned to calm as swiftly as it had turned to anger. 'Bastard.' She spat the words out and Laura could hear the venom being released as she did so.

'Yeah, you don't want the bastard fucking you up anymore.'

'No.' There was a silence. 'I'm feeling very sleepy. I'll go now, and I will see you next week, I promise. I'm so sorry. Please forgive me, I really will make it next week.'

'Nothing to forgive, Jennifer, nothing to forgive. I look forward to seeing you next week.' Laura knew she meant it as she spoke these words. She totally accepted Jennifer's choice to drink to cope. She felt fully and completely OK with the choice that Jennifer had made, although she was sorry that she had needed to use alcohol. But when you are hurt and confused and desperate to feel different, and you know there is a magic potion in a bottle or a can that will do just that, it's bloody difficult not to use it.

'Thank you. See you next week.'

Laura heard the clunk of the phone being put down. She slowly returned the receiver herself and went back into the counselling room to sit down and be with her thoughts. Oh well, she thought, it's going to be difficult. She thought of Jennifer and what she must be going through, and her thoughts drifted to the many women, and men, all over the world who had suffered sexual abuse in childhood and who were struggling to cope with the memories and the emotional and psychological effects that rippled into their lives. Ripple. Stupid word to use. Often it wasn't just a ripple, more of a tidal wave banking up in the depths of a person's oceanic self, waiting to break out dramatically on the shore of awareness. It took her mind back to a book she had read, Sanderson's *Counselling Adult Survivors of Child Sexual Abuse*, which gives such a useful account of the effects.

So many effects. And so many people used substances to blot it all out, or at least try to. She knew that not everyone did, but the numbers who drank to cope with memories, or the traumatised emotions, were high. She shook her head. And then there are all those children who are being sexually abused now, she thought to herself, in this moment, now, as I sit here. She closed her eyes. What a world we have created. She could feel so many emotions herself, anger, sadness, helplessness in the face of the vastness of the problem. I can't heal everyone, I can't take this terrible experience away from people, but I can try to help those who come to me. And at least I am not alone, there are many more like me trying to help people to come to terms with their pain and confusion.

She quietly wrote her notes about the telephone contact with Jennifer and slowly, and what would have appeared quite reverently, placed them back in her filing cabinet. She turned, took another look around the room, turned off the light and closed the door behind her.

Supervision

'I need some time on Jennifer. It's all coming back and she's drinking again. And I feel very affected by it all. I haven't been able to put it aside since I spoke to Jennifer a couple of evenings ago when she hadn't made it to her appointment. She's in a bad way, very fragile, very desperate, but still determined to come through. And it seems her partner is really supportive, and that must be huge for her.' The words came out quite rapidly, the result of being bottled up since the telephone conversation.

Malcolm was struck by the intensity of what Laura was saying and wondered how it was impacting on her own wellbeing and inner feelings. It seemed to be quite overwhelming. 'Where do you want to start, Laura? And I'm really wondering how you are in all of this.'

'I feel for her, Malcolm, I really feel for her. It all came out, well, not all, she doesn't seem to have clear memories yet, well, I assume not though I don't know. I mean, that had happened when I last saw her and it didn't get mentioned on the telephone. I guess I don't know. But she knows she was sexually abused. In the session after she got back from holiday she flipped into a younger self, not the

7-year-old, but younger, and she talked about the games she played with daddy. She talked about how he let her touch him, well, encouraged her to touch him, and he touched her. She said that, and this was horrible to hear, she said that she was touching his worm and that it was a friendly worm. But then she said that it bit her and hurt her. What the hell was he doing to her? She didn't say. The 7-year-old part of her cut in. And whilst these parts of her were speaking, Jennifer was listening but not in a place to say anything. She could only listen to what was being said, what she was saying. It was awful. She broke down immediately that she came back to her adult self. The pain, the hurt, the shock. I just held her and held her whilst she cried and clung to me. I mean, I'm so glad that she was able to release all this feeling, but it was so, so intense. I feel drained talking about it. And she was absolutely wiped out at the end of the session, had to call her partner to come and pick her up. She didn't feel safe to drive.' Laura could feel herself becoming progressively more tired. Her eyes felt really heavy.

'You look so tired, Laura.'

'I can hardly keep my eyes open. I wasn't feeling this way when I came in, but talking about Jennifer. I feel so tired.'

'Tired of?'

'No, just tired.' Laura closed her eyes.

'What are you experiencing within the tiredness?' Laura could hear Malcolm's question but it seemed distant. She could feel herself drifting off. 'Heavy, very heavy. Weighted down. Unable to move.'

Laura suddenly felt herself clearing and she opened her eyes.

'What is it?'

'Weighted down, heavy. Jennifer described herself as feeling paralysed after realising what had happened, unable to move.'

Malcolm thought back to his telephone contact with Jennifer. 'In the conversation I had with her when she called me while you were away, she talked about pressure on her chest, I'm sure she did. Or am I mistaken? In a dream or something, waking up, feeling pressure on her body. No, I responded with the words "pressure on her body", she had spoken about pressure on her chest. But after I had said those words she went very quiet on me on the phone. Something happened but she didn't really know what. She spoke of feeling distant, small, not really herself.' Malcolm brought his thoughts back to Laura. 'How are you feeling now?'

'I have woken up. I feel more connected somehow.'

'More connected?'

'Yes, something has shifted and it is perhaps around this sense of Jennifer feeling paralysed, and now hearing what you are saying, it starts to make sense. But it is a connection that Jennifer has not made yet, isn't it?'

Malcolm heard what Laura was saying. 'No, she hasn't, and you say that she doesn't have any clear memories yet of exactly what happened?'

'No, but the dreams that had been upsetting her, they ... of course, she would have been laying down in bed. Perhaps lying down is loosening up memories. Or rather, leaving her reliving physical sensations.' Laura brought her hand up to her mouth as she thought about what she had said.

'What is it?'

'I don't know. It's like I feel really close to something but can't grasp what it is.'

'Think you are parallel processing somehow with Jennifer?'

Parallel processing is where a feature of the client's experiencing is played out within someone else. In this case, the fact that Jennifer is no doubt carrying memories but has not yet connected with them is being paralleled in Laura's process of feeling that something is present but feeling unable to connect with it. Laura's tiredness and heaviness could also be seen as a similar phenomenon. It can be useful to identify and work with as it can often shed light on what may be present for the client, or on incongruent elements within the counsellor that could block accurate empathy.

'Yes. I have a strong sense that Jennifer is on the edge of a lot of memories and I really feel for her and can so understand that part of her wants to keep well away from it and I guess the alcohol is part of that. But we know alcohol can also release feelings as well, and I hope that when memories and feelings do come back that they are at a time when she can deal with them.'

'Sounds like you don't trust her process?'

Laura shook her head. 'No, not when there's a chemical involved. The alcohol could disinhibit and release feelings she might not be able to contain. Or she might react to it all alcohol-affected and do something she might regret, like, well maybe talk to someone in the family when she hasn't really thought through what she wants to say or when she wants to say it.' Laura paused. 'But then maybe she already has, I don't know. And, of course, we know the depressant affect of alcohol and the suicide risk. I don't sense that to be present, but alcohol and depression can be such a lethal cocktail.'

Malcolm was aware he was still carrying his earlier question. 'Yes. But you are not sensing that it is triggering that kind of reaction?'

'No, but if there is a part of her that is self-abusing . . . . Oh shit, she accidently cut herself a while back – you don't suppose that was a self-abusing part of herself? And the drinking might be linked into self-abuse, although it seems more likely it is connected to the need to just blot out and anaesthetise – as though it is a way of killing memories. I just hope that I can continue to help the parts of her that need to find their voice to do so, and hope that some other part of herself doesn't try to take over and stop the voices permanently.'

'Sounds like it has become more of a real concern as you have been speaking?'

'I need to be aware of this. And I mustn't let my anxiety based on all this speculation get in the way of hearing what Jennifer needs to tell me when I see her next. She needs me to be focused and empathic, and she needs a lot of unconditional warmth. She needs a lot of love, doesn't she, real love. I hope that she experiences this with Ian and it doesn't start to get conditional on her being a certain way. That will just feed back into the effects of the abuse.'

'I want to acknowledge what you are saying and part of me is still with the question of how you are with it all, Laura. How is it affecting you as a counsellor, as a person, as a woman?'

She shuddered. 'That was a response to the "as a woman". Something that has been with me since that session, although it didn't strike me at the time, is that I don't remember all of my childhood. Do any of us? Jennifer didn't and suddenly she is being confronted with memories emerging from within herself that she simply was not aware of. So where does that leave us, me? It just makes you think.'

'Makes you think, yeah.'

'I'm pretty sure I didn't experience abuse as a child, sexual or otherwise. And I have to live to that belief, but hearing Jennifer makes me realise it is a belief, I don't actually know that I was never the victim of sexual abuse in childhood. And isn't that what we all believe, unless we have memories or something specific to tell us different? I guess it has reinforced for me that you have to be ready for the unexpected all the time, yet not to the point that it gets in the way of getting on with life. So that's part of my reaction. I also felt a tremendous sense of solidarity with Jennifer when I was holding her, it really felt like a merging and it felt like it was a real woman-to-woman experience. That was powerful for me, like we connected at some deep level where there was no need for words, there was a shared experience of the presence of pain.' As she spoke Laura could feel her eyes watering and emotions rising within her. 'Really gets to me.' Tears began to flow. Laura took a tissue and wiped her eyes. 'It's good to be affected, tells me my feelings are engaging in this process. I need them. I'd hate to feel I was detached. I need to be in there, and I really did feel it that way. Jennifer needs to experience a person, and maybe a woman, hearing what she is going through, a person with feelings and thoughts, who is human and vulnerable like she is.'

'It is expected that the relationship with the therapist is the meeting of two live, real human beings, with the therapist fully present to his client. This situation is at the furthest pole from the therapist as an expert, analyzing the patient as object. It is a living together in communication that breaks the isolation of the patient' (Rogers, 1959, p. 197).

'A lot of thoughts and feelings there, not sure which thread you want to pick up on, but I really heard that sense of deep solidarity and the importance to you of being affected by your clients, and by Jennifer.' Malcolm also appreciated the importance of being affected by clients, of being very much in, rather than apart from, the therapeutic process. He saw it as central to effective therapy, part of the process of meeting person to person.

It is OK for a counsellor to be tearful and affected by a client. It is a genuine response. It is not regarded as an issue if a counsellor should feel good and express it if a client is in celebratory mood, so why not when a client is sad or in distress. So long as the essential fact that the counsellor is there for the

> client is not lost sight of, the person-centred counsellor will want to bring their authentic self into the relationship with the client.

'I think it was the effect of Jennifer talking as a child, it made it so much more vivid, made a greater impression on me. Whatever did it do to her, though? No wonder she is struggling at the moment. I really want to scoop that little girl up, hug her, protect her and tell her it is alright. I know that's partly a mothering instinct, but it feels more than that. It's back to that sense of solidarity, and yet I know that I'm not anti-men and I don't want to get into feeling that is what it is about. I don't think it is. I've explored that in the past. No, it's . . . .' Laura thought for a moment. 'No, it's like, well, I'm thinking of my sister's daughter now, how I'd want to stand with my sister to be there for her daughter. Not that she's been abused but, it's something like that. It's, yes, it's a kind of sisterhood thing.'

Malcolm nodded, aware that as a man he was not privy to that sense and yet he had experienced being at men's workshops and had felt a gender solidarity in those settings which had been incredibly powerful. And he had been to workshops where he was the only man and had felt very much a part, probably because he had what some termed a 'strong feminine side'. 'It sounds profound to experience sisterhood.'

'It is, and yet maybe it is also something of an adult thing as well, you know, wanting to reach out to children who are vulnerable or hurting. I also feel good about working with Jennifer, you know, I really want to help her and I believe that the relationship we have built over the months has created something that will enable her to come through this. No, that's too grandiose, but it will help and support her in finding *her* way through it.'

'Seems to me that the relationship you have with her has created the opportunity for all this to emerge.'

'Yes, I think you are right.'

'So it says something about the effectiveness of the work you are doing with Jennifer, Laura, what a good therapist you are.'

'Thanks. I think I need to hear that.' She felt emotion and she smiled. She nodded her head, 'Yeah, I need to hear that.'

Malcolm did not interrupt the silence that followed for a while. He sensed the importance of allowing Laura to be with and to absorb her feelings and thoughts around being a good therapist. Finally, after Laura had smiled again and nodded, he continued.

'Anything else you want to explore about your feelings towards Jennifer?'

Laura thought for a moment. She knew she was a little apprehensive, no be honest, she was apprehensive as to what was going to emerge in the coming months and she also felt good to be there for her client. 'I feel apprehensive but also good. It is going to be challenging and I am sure it is going to move me in many ways. I want to be able to be myself and be with Jennifer in all of this. I feel I can fully accept her. I may get angry towards her father at times, I am sure I will, and I will need to resolve that here if it gets in the way of my empathising with Jennifer. But I feel good about it. The past has happened and Jennifer has a life ahead of her. I really want to help her claim the life that she wants. Yeah, I feel good about that.' Laura could feel quite a surge of energy as she said those last few words – Jennifer claiming a life for herself, yes, that felt like what it was all about.

Points for discussion

- What has contributed to enabling Jennifer to disclose her experience as a child?
- What would your concerns be if a client was to regress into a much younger state within the session?
- Evaluate how Laura handled the disclosure?
- What are the issues to consider when a client is feeling unable to make their own way home at the end of the session?
- How would you react to a client not turning up to a session because they had been drinking?
- Did you feel that the telephone conversation offered enough support and encouragement to Jennifer? Would you have responded differently and, if so, how?
- Do you feel that Laura brought all the pertinent issues to supervision, or if you had been Laura were there other factors that you would have wanted to explore?
- What implications and issues may have arisen if Laura had been a male counsellor in session 37?

CHAPTER 6

Counselling session 39

It was 7.30pm precisely when the doorbell rang and Laura went to let Jennifer in.
'Hi.' Laura smiled as she looked at Jennifer.
'Hi. I'm really sorry about last week, really sorry.'
'That's OK, come on through. It must have been an awful time for you.'
'Yes.' Jennifer took off her coat and sat down.
'So. Where do you want to start this evening?' Laura wanted to keep it completely
    open and to give Jennifer the freedom to find her own direction once again. She
    hoped it conveyed her trust in Jennifer's process.
'I don't know really. I feel as though I am still trying to make sense of everything,
    and I'm afraid that the drinking just got out of control. It really did. I ended up
    seeing my GP on Friday and he prescribed me tranquillisers, partly to settle me
    down a bit and partly to help me stop the alcohol. They've helped, but I haven't
    started to cut them back like he said I should, and I am going to run out so I
    need to speak to him again. Anyway, I'll deal with that. I know I can't rely on
    them, but they have helped. But I do feel strange. As though I'm only partly
    feeling things. Weird, but I think I needed it.'
'It really did get away from you then but you are finding the tranquillisers are
    helping. And I hear your concern that you are taking too many.'
'Yes. I stopped the alcohol on Saturday. It was getting crazy. I had got up to two
    bottles a night when I phoned you, I'd had the first and had the second after
    talking to you. Thursday I had half a bottle of vodka and I knew then I had to
    do something. Haven't had spirits in months, and I know that it just does my
    head in. I told the GP what had happened, it wasn't easy, but I knew I had to.
    And he was good. He said he appreciated that I had tried to tranquillise myself
    on alcohol and that if he prescribed me something it would be more controlled.
    So, here I am, dry but only half feeling anything.'
'It's helpful to know that, as I might be confused by feeling you were disengaging
    from your feelings, or might think it is part of your own process of dealing with
    the situation rather than a chemical effect. So, drinking has stopped, tranquil-
    lisers are working, feeling weird.'

'And I'm getting some strange thoughts in my head, and images that I can't really
make sense of, or at least, I guess I can but I suppose I'm afraid to. And anyway,
it's weird, I think things and see things but I don't have feelings about them.
I guess that's the tranquillisers. It's like watching a scary movie without feeling
scared. In a way it's good, but I know it can't last.'

'Thoughts and images but no feelings.' Laura kept her response brief, holding the
focus on the essence of what Jennifer was saying. She made a mental note that
it was probably pointless to try to hold Jennifer on feelings this session. But
that didn't mean the session couldn't be useful. She would still be empathic to
what Jennifer was experiencing. Anyway, there was more to counselling than
feelings, although she also realised that Jennifer's inability to be in touch with
her own experiencing was significant.

Working with a client who is affected by medication, particularly tranquillisers, can leave the counsellor feeling strangely detached from the client and
struggling to feel a connection, although the fact that there is an interaction
and that the client is aware of the counsellor's presence will mean that contact is present.

'I still see my father's face and I have figured out when it was. I would have been
about five, maybe four, I was at school in the day and came home I suppose
about 3.00pm. Mum collected me, my sister was with her. She was two or
three. We had tea when we came home. My father came in from work and I
think I was with him when my mother bathed my sister. I think that's what
was happening. But before I was six my father took a job overseas for a year.
By then my sister was starting school as well and so my mother coped with us.
So I guess it started when I was four or five.'

'So you think it started when you were four or five and your father went overseas
before you were six?' Laura was aware of how calm Jennifer seemed, although
her voice was a little weak and shaky. It was the emotion that was missing.

Jennifer nodded, slowly. 'I still don't remember exactly what happened though.
Can't seem to get that, but something must be there after what I heard myself
saying last time. Funny, I don't seem to go into that state anywhere else.'

'Mmmm, only here.'

'Yes. And I wonder why it all started to happen now, I mean, why now? And why
can't I remember it all?'

Laura heard her inner voice respond with 'because the time is right but not right
for everything' but didn't want to give Jennifer answers she might well need to
unravel for herself. She simply reflected back Jennifer's question. 'Why can't I
remember it all?'

'I guess something is keeping it back, and I suppose the only something is me.'

'So something in you is controlling what you become aware of, is that what you
are saying?'

'I guess so. But why did it start now? What started it all off. It seemed that I was fine, doing really well, wasn't I? We were talking about ending the counselling not so long ago. God, that seems a million miles away now, and even further with these drugs!' She smiled weakly. Laura smiled back.

'Yes, they can have that effect. We were talking about ending, then what happened?' Laura posed the question as clearly this was an issue Jennifer was wrestling with.

'I went to my sister's. That was OK. Then things started to feel not right somehow, disturbed, and I . . . when did I pass out?'

Laura thought about it. 'The week before you went to your sister's, I think. I'm not one hundred per cent sure, but I think it was then.'

'OK. And then I went away and we had a good time and I came back. And I was feeling troubled. I remember, was it the next session or the session afterwards, I really did not feel good and was looking at the clock. But I didn't know why.'

'Mmmm, that's how I remember it.' Laura said nothing else, leaving Jennifer freedom to continue to reflect on her process.

Laura could have empathised with the 'But I didn't know why', but has rather chosen to empathise with the context of Jennifer wanting to reflect over the process through the sessions. This kind of decision has to be made sometimes and it is easy for the counsellor to not even be aware that they have made a choice that directs the client's focus. Laura is centred in her own remembering process and has stepped out of the client's frame of reference.

'And there was that long silence, and I didn't know what had happened. And that was something new to me. So that was after something must have triggered me, or caused that sense of unease to start to emerge.' Jennifer shook her head and yawned. 'God it's difficult to concentrate at the moment. My head feels as though it is full of cotton wool, all fuzzy and clogged up somehow.' She blinked a few times, trying to regain her focus but it was very difficult. 'Don't think I should have driven over tonight. I'll have to be very careful going back. The tablets should have worn off a bit by then, I last took one at six o'clock.'

Laura felt a need to know what she was taking and how much so she could gauge the likely effect.

'Can I just ask what you are taking and how much?'

'Yes, diazepam, what else! One 5 milligram tablet four times a day. Should have reduced it down to two tablets by now, but that will have to wait.'

Laura noted this in her mind, and realised that yes, this could well be having a strong effect. She knew that different people reacted differently, different levels of sensitivity. She knew that if she took that amount she would be flat out, having a very low tolerance threshold for a lot of medications. She also knew that Jennifer might find it easier to reduce if she switched to 2 mg tablets. Not everyone was aware of this and having remembered it herself she felt it appropriate to share it. 'Before we continue I just want to say that it can be prescribed in 2 mg tablets and that can make it easier to cut back in smaller amounts. Just wanted you to be aware of that option, but I don't want this bit of info cutting across your focus.'

Information can run the risk of the counsellor assuming some expert posi-tion, which is not what the person-centred approach is about. However, when a counsellor has information that might be helpful to the client it does not seem to be an act of unconditional positive regard to withhold it. The appropriateness of giving information is governed largely by motive. If it is an expression of warmth and concern for the client, and is not an attempt to tell the client what is best for them, then it is more likely to be helpful and less likely to undermine the person-centred therapeutic alliance.

'Thanks, I hadn't realised that. Makes a lot of sense.' Jennifer was really grateful that Laura had taken the trouble to point this out.

'OK. So, you were struggling to get hold of what triggered the unease?'

'Yeah, but it seems to point to the trip southwest.'

'Mmmm. So, what was it about that trip?' Jennifer spoke slowly.

Laura sat quietly and allowed Jennifer the space to think. Lots of different images were coming up for Jennifer as she reflected back on that trip. The meal out, the trips to the beach, so many images passed through her mind as she reflected. It had felt good, being together again as a family, sharing the time. Another memory came into Jennifer's mind. 'Oh SHIT.' Laura noticed Jennifer going pale. 'Oh my God. Oh no. Oh Sweet Jesus no.' Jennifer could feel the horror rising up inside herself. Her parents had come down and were staying in a cot-tage nearby. They had been at the birthday party. Susie's birthday party. Jen-nifer could feel the goose bumps breaking out all over her body, her arms, legs, up her neck.

Laura could see the look of horror that had broken out on Jennifer's face and she felt she could have cut the atmosphere with a knife. It was electric.

'What is it, Jennifer, what have you remembered?'

'My father . . . my father was there. He had Susie on his lap. Oh God, no, I've got to phone my sister.'

'What happened Jennifer?'

'The look on his face. I've seen that look before. It's the one I keep seeing, I see in my dreams.' She looked up at Laura. 'Oh God, Laura, what do I do? Jennifer closed her eyes and breathed deeply, bringing her hand up to her face as she did so. She shivered. 'What do I do? It's happening again.' Jennifer just hadn't thought about that. She had been so convinced in herself that she had been the only victim.

It is not unusual for survivors of child sexual abuse to believe that they are their abuser's only victim. This is partly because they might be thinking that perhaps they were protecting another sibling by taking it themselves, or because they are still carrying an internalised belief that they are 'special' to the abuser.

Laura wanted to empathise with Jennifer yet she was also aware that the look she saw on her father's face did not necessarily mean what Jennifer was thinking, particularly as that expression clearly had been associated with traumatic experiencing in her own life.

'I hear your concern, Jennifer, but are you sure it is happening again?' Laura knew she had stepped out of Jennifer's world. She quickly sought to step back in it. 'You want to do something but don't know what.'

Jennifer had heard Laura doubting her, or at least that's what it had felt like. It made her feel strangely anxious, which was weird through the tranquillised haze. 'I know that look, Laura, I know it. I've seen it before. It's vivid. I know it. Oh God, it's going to rip the family apart.' Jennifer paused and it appeared as though a new worry had passed into her facial expression. 'What if they don't believe me, Laura, it happens? No one believes you. I haven't said anything yet, I nearly did, I wanted to but Ian stopped me. I was glad he did, I don't think I would have handled it well when I was drinking. But Laura, I've got to do something. It was that which must have troubled me, but I didn't know why. But it must have touched something deep. Brought . . . oh, it's no good speculating on that, I've got to do something. Oh God. It's got worse and I still haven't remembered exactly what happened to me.' Jennifer put her head in her hands and shook her head again.

'What do you want to do, Jennifer?' Laura spoke slowly and softly, trying to create a reflective atmosphere.

'I don't know. Do I confront my father? Do I talk to my sister? Do I . . . what other options have I got? I've got to do something.'

'OK, I hear you really clearly, you feel you've got to do something. I have to say that we have to consider the safety of Susie first and foremost here, yes?'

'Yes. So I need to speak to my sister, don't I? She has to know first. It'll shatter her world. But I have to. I have to, I can't not talk to her, tell her. I need to explain what has happened here, don't I? I need to talk her through what I have been experiencing. And then I guess we have to make a decision together.'

The thought passed through Laura's mind that Jennifer was making a huge assumption that Susie was at risk, but more than that, she was assuming that if Susie was at risk of, or was a victim of sexual abuse from Jennifer's father, it was only contained within the family. Oh shit, Laura thought, Jennifer isn't thinking of that, but she probably needs to. Her head was racing with thoughts and she had to slow it down. She took a deep breath.

Laura has left Jennifer's frame of reference but has realised and slows herself down, giving Jennifer the choice as to which direction she wishes to take the session in.

'OK, we have a choice to explore your feelings, explore your options, explore the implications of your father as a sexual abuser of little girls.' God, that sounded awful as she said it, and she immediately realised that it should feel awful, it was awful, but she needed to hold her focus and let Jennifer work through what she needed to address. This was Jennifer's process, she, Laura, could take her own reactions to supervision.

Jennifer nodded. Hearing Laura speak really stopped her in her tracks. This was the horror of it, staring her in the face. Her father, a sexual abuser of little girls. Little girls. Oh no, what if . . . ? She looked at Laura and Laura knew what Jennifer was thinking. She nodded her head without saying a word.

'I have to speak to my sister tonight, when I get back. OK, I'm clear on that, and we have to confront him, we have to. I've woken up, Laura, the haze in my head has cleared, at least for now. Must be adrenalin release. My heart is pounding. OK, speak to my sister, hear what she thinks. Oh God, my sister. You don't suppose . . . ? And she might be like me, blanked it all out. No, I've got to see her, face to face. I can't talk on the phone. I have to go down and see her. She's going to need me, and, we're going to need each other. Oh what an absolute nightmare. Part of me feels like I'm going to explode, but I mustn't. I . . . OK, I'm clear what I have to do.'

Laura felt good that Jennifer had reached a decision and it was her own decision. She felt it was realistic. 'OK, clear what you have to do?'

'Yes, I'll call her this evening when I get back. No, I'd better talk to Ian first, he needs to know as he'll want to come down. I'll have to cancel my hair appointment and maybe we can get away on Friday if we can get time off. Damn, that means I need to see the GP tomorrow. I'll have to explain it all to him if I can get past the receptionist.'

Laura listened as Jennifer continued to think out loud what she had to do. What a roller coaster she was on. She noticed Jennifer look at the clock, although there was plenty of time left in the session. 'Look, I think I need to head off, start getting things organised, make phone calls.'

'You need to do what is most pressing, Jennifer, and I guess at this precise moment counselling is not on the top of the list. So please, head off. Do what you need to do. It sounds as though you have made some decisions and others will flow out of talking to your sister. Part of me would like to offer you space to think that through, but I also realise that maybe that isn't your priority at this moment.' I'm talking too much, Laura thought, I guess I'm picking up on the anxiety and I'm babbling. Slow down.

There was a lot of anxious energy being released, and Jennifer cannot contain her need to take action and start to organise seeing her sister. She isn't going to stay and process her experience, and Laura empathises with this and accepts Jennifer's need to act. She also recognises that she is being swept up by it all and is taking steps to slow her reaction. Where this is happening it can be difficult to genuinely empathise, or for the client to really hear what the therapist is saying. The internal process takes over, all the action is taking place within Jennifer and it is difficult, if not impossible, for her to hear or receive anything coming in from outside. Allowing her to head off – the client is surely free so is it a matter of allowing? – might be regarded as an example of empathy towards the context, or 'situational empathy'.

'No, I'll be OK. I feel focused. I need to head off. I feel as though I've reached a place today that requires me to take action. So I'll see you next week, same time, yes?' Jennifer had put on her coat and had opened the door. Laura followed her out.

'Yes. Good luck with everything, Jennifer, I will be thinking of you. We'll talk it through next week.' Jennifer had opened the door and was heading out.

'I think I'm going to have a lot to talk through next week.' With that Jennifer turned away and headed down the path. 'Thanks. See you next week.'

'Bye. Take care.' And she was gone through the gate and behind the hedge to where her car was parked.

Laura closed the door. 'Be prepared for anything', that should be written above all counselling doors. She went into the kitchen and took a grapefruit juice from the fridge. It tasted cold and refreshing. She walked back into the counselling room and sat down and thought back over the session. Had she handled it OK? This was getting very serious and she thought of the legal side of it all. She kept her notes clear, concise and factual. She then got out another piece of paper and began to jot down her own thoughts and feelings, not with any particular plan, just as they came. It felt like a release, just noting down her speculations and concerns. Laura found it helpful on occasions and this was one of those occasions.

Counselling session 40

After settling into the session and saying a little bit about her day at work – it had been extremely hectic and had left Jennifer feeling tired and listless – she began to talk about the weekend with her sister. She explained how they had driven down on the Friday afternoon and arrived early evening, having stopped on the way for a couple of breaks as the motorway had been awful with really heavy rain and spray. The journey had taken longer than they had expected.

'I wasn't really sure what to say or how to say it, but I knew I had to get things out in the open.'

'Mmmm, can't have been easy.' Laura responded as much to the situation as to the tone of Jennifer's voice, which sounded hesitant and a little constrained.

'No, it wasn't.' Jennifer paused for a while. 'But I did bring it up, after we had eaten a meal. I said that I wanted some time alone with Angie as I felt I needed to talk to her sister-to-sister. I mean, I knew that Ian was aware, but I really wanted to talk to her alone. I didn't know what she was going to say and having Ian in the room and maybe her husband, John, might have made it awkward. Anyway, we actually went and sat in the kitchen. I told her what had happened in my counselling and how I was making sense of it. I told her how shocked I was, and how hard it had been to accept and yet I realised I had to. I didn't say more than that to begin with. I didn't want to start scaring her about her daughter.'

Laura nodded and said nothing as she wanted to leave her to continue with her story. Jennifer knew she was listening.

'Angie sat there looking at me across the table and was shaking her head, saying "No, not Dad, oh God, no, are you sure, I mean, are you really sure?" I said that I could only tell her what I had experienced, that I hadn't got clear memories of anything actually happening, but that I had begun to remember about the fear waiting for him to come home, and his face in the dreams and that awful sense of pressure and weight on my body.' Jennifer looked down as she finished and remained silent for a few moments. Laura respected her silence. It was clearly not easy for Jennifer to describe what had happened. 'She told me that she couldn't remember that age, that she didn't know. She asked me how I could be so sure. I said that somehow, something deep in me seemed to know that what I heard myself saying was true. I told her how I had been drinking again and was trying to bring it back under control, but how difficult the evenings were.' Jennifer looked up. 'We ended up hugging and crying. She believed me, Laura, you don't know what a relief that was. I really didn't know. I mean, we get on well now, but I really did not know how she was going to react. But she believed me, thank goodness. I don't know what I would have done if she didn't believe me. Yes I do. I'd have gone out, or back home, and got drunk.'

'Real relief, a real relief at being believed.'

'Yes.' Jennifer let out a long slow breath. There were tears in her eyes. 'I don't think I've ever felt as close to my sister as I did that evening. It was so good. After we had talked I felt utterly drained, I mean, I just couldn't keep my eyes open. We decided to call it a night, but I said I wanted to talk more the next day. Anyway, I went up and had a bath. Ian came up a little while later. He said that Angie had told him about the conversation we had just had and that she was going to tell John. Ian left them to talk about it and came up to me. You know, I got through that evening without a drink, well, we had a glass with the meal but there was just the one bottle between the four of us, so it was hardly a drink really, not what I usually have.'

'Felt good about getting through with just the glass.'

'Yes. And then Ian and I talked for a little, but not long. We were both tired and we soon fell asleep. Didn't get a chance to say anything more the next morning. The children wanted to go out and we decided to go up to the coast. Went for a walk, had lunch out and tried to enjoy ourselves, but I guess we were all feeling a bit subdued.' Jennifer added a little more about what they did and then went on to the evening. 'We started talking again after dinner, the children were in bed. I knew I had to say something. So I said what I was concerned about and how I'd seen that look on my dad's face. John just exploded. He was so angry. Never seen him like that, we had to hold him back from phoning my father then and there. He wanted to call the police, ended up drinking too much himself, he was so upset. It was only later that I heard that he'd had a rough time as a child and that he is always badly affected when he hears about children being hurt.'

Jennifer drank more water. 'It was awful. None of us knew what to do. Then the door opened and Jack came in – he couldn't sleep. Angie took him back up. Somehow that made a difference. When Angie came back down we had agreed we had to confront my father, and Angie agreed as well. "But what about Mum?" We all turned to Angie and realised that none of us knew what to say. We decided we needed to talk to him alone. Angie phoned him and we are going to visit him this weekend. The idea is that we tell Mum that we want a chat with Dad and John is going to take her out with the children – she gets on well with John, and Ian will go with them. We'll meet up beforehand so we can arrive together.' Jennifer took in a deep breath. 'So that's where it's at now. I'm not looking forward to it, but it has to happen.'

Laura nodded. Jennifer sensed from the expression on Laura's face that she had heard what she had been saying. She didn't want her to respond, but continued, changing the subject.

Laura has had to say very little. Clients sometimes simply need to tell their story and they do not want to be interrupted with constant reflections, or have something summarised that it is not important for them to hear back from their counsellor. Jennifer doesn't want to explore what she has been saying, but rather say it to inform Laura as to what happened. Having done that, she moves on.

'I've been having more memories as well. I had another long chat with my sister on the Sunday, the men took the children out in the morning. She told me she had never understood why my mother had always seen her as the favourite, but wondered if she knew and blamed me. She said she had no recollection of any kind of abuse herself, but she did remember that Dad gave me more attention. She had always felt jealous, now she felt guilty. I said I still didn't really know what had happened, but I felt strongly that something did.'

'Strong feeling, yeah?'

'It is, but it feels weird, like I know something but don't know what it is. But it's there and it feels so heavy and draining, and I'm feeling more anxious. The GP switched me to 2 mg tablets but I haven't been able to reduce. Then on Monday night I had a really awful dream, woke up screaming. Didn't know why but I felt as though I was – this'll sound crazy – I felt as though I wasn't me, at least, felt as though I was outside of myself. I mean, looking at myself somehow. Felt scary. Felt like I couldn't get back, that was the nightmare. I wasn't in my body and I couldn't get back into it. Shit, I was sweating and . . . I felt awful, really shaky. Took me ages to settle again. Ian tried to calm me down but there was something really vivid about that dream, well, it was a nightmare really. Haven't been able to get rid of that sense of being out of myself. I mean, it's still with me now, I can easily relive it, as though it is really close.'

Laura nodded. 'So, feeling that you were kind of out of your body and terrified you couldn't get back, and you can still feel those feelings, even now?'

'Yes.' Jennifer could feel herself trembling. 'I'm going mad, aren't I?'

'You think you're going mad, Jennifer?'

'Yes,' there was a pause, 'and no. I mean, oh, I don't know. Just feels very, very unsettling, you know. I don't want it again, but I do think about it, well, I did last night, and I guess I will tonight. I drank a bit more last night. Took a while to get to sleep but I did in the end.'

'Mmmm. Hard to get to sleep with this on your mind.'

Jennifer went silent and it lasted a couple of minutes. She was very much in her own thoughts, and finally she looked up. 'There's going to be more, isn't there? This is just the beginning, isn't it?'

Laura was mindful of not wanting to encourage any beliefs and therefore expectations in Jennifer. She kept her response simple, seeking to convey that she had heard Jennifer's wondering. 'You feel that there's more?'

Jennifer just nodded in response, and reached for a tissue. She could feel a kind of deep, tired sadness welling up inside herself and a sense of coldness. She shivered. 'I think there's more. But I don't want to start looking for it. I know I have to get on with my life as best I can and I guess be prepared for more memories to surface.' She went on to ask if Laura thought that the nightmare had anything to do with it. Laura didn't confirm her own thoughts, but encouraged Jennifer to air hers. She said she thought it did. She was feeling very tired. She hadn't really got over the weekend, and then that sleepless night last night with the nightmare. The tiredness grew.

She could feel tension in her body, her shoulders were tight, her back ached and she could also feel a tightness in her thighs. Somehow her body felt different, as though she was stretched, the tight points seemed distant from each other. She could feel her shoulders and her back but they somehow seemed a long way away from her legs, and particularly her thighs. It was as though she was detached from them. They seemed to feel further and further away as she felt herself drifting with the tiredness. It was a strange feeling, unsettling but she had no energy to feel much about it.

'That was weird.'

'Weird?'

'I could feel a real tension in my legs, in my thighs and I seemed to feel suddenly very distant from them. I mean, like I was up here,' Jennifer lifted her hands up to her head and waved them in front of her face, upper chest and shoulders, 'and down here,' she touched her thighs, 'was somehow far away.' Jennifer shook her head and looked puzzled.

'Like you were centred in your upper body but your thighs were distant in some way?' Laura empathised with a question, inviting a further response and clarification as she wasn't completely sure what Jennifer was meaning.

'Like I was separated, somehow, yes, separated more than distant.' She shivered. 'Somehow made me think of that nightmare again. Don't know what that's about.'

'The separation makes you think of the nightmare.'

Jennifer was silent again. 'I don't understand but it doesn't feel good.' She lifted her hands to her mouth and her eyes seemed to Laura to open a little wider.

'Doesn't feel good . . . .'

Jennifer shook her head. 'No.' She still felt very tired, and she glanced at the clock. Laura noticed the glance and looked as well. A few minutes left.

'Yes, I think I need to head off and get some sleep. I need an early night. I hope I don't have that nightmare again. I really do.'

'That nightmare really has affected you deeply, hasn't it?'

Jennifer nodded. 'Yes, it was and is so vivid.' She took a deep breath and blew it out slowly. 'Yes, it's vivid.'

'Vivid.'

Jennifer nodded. 'And the weird thing is as I sit here thinking about it, I want to say that it's somehow familiar, but I don't remember ever having any kind of experience like this. But then, there are lots of things I don't seem to be remembering. Oh well, I just have to keep on going and see what happens. And I've got to get myself together for Saturday. That's the big thing now. I hope it doesn't go badly, but I don't know what to expect, I don't really know what I want to happen. I mean, maybe he might admit to it, but he might deny it. He might get angry. I just don't know. I just don't know.'

'That sounds scary, the "I just don't know".'

'Yes, don't know what I'm preparing myself for, but I am going to tell him and I know that Angie wants to know. We have to know. We can't have Susie at risk. John is really clear. Any doubt and that's it, no contact with Susie. And if it comes to that then we will have to explain it to Mum. But we'll see. Never thought I'd be faced with this, Laura, other people, not me. But it is me and I have to face it. And whatever else emerges.' She paused, looked at the clock, and added, 'OK, time to head off. I need the fresh air as well I think, wake me up a bit.' She yawned again. 'Oh dear, I will drive carefully.'

They agreed the same time next week and Jennifer left. Laura wrote up her notes and reflected on how she was feeling. The out-of-body dream was not unusual. Lots of people had out-of-body experiences, and some of them were linked to the experience of child sexual abuse. But she didn't want to make the connection for Jennifer, she must make this herself, and she felt sure that memories would begin to surface. Too many things were happening. A process was running for Jennifer and it was highly likely that the parts of herself that were associated with the sexual abuse were becoming closer to Jennifer's normal waking awareness.

Counselling session 41

Jennifer attended the following week and spent most of the session talking about the confrontation she and her sister had had with her father. She was angry and upset in the session. Her father had denied it had happened, saying it was rubbish and that her therapist was putting ideas in her head, that he was her father, that he loved her and that he would never have done such a thing. Jennifer had been left feeling angry and confused. She did not believe him but she had not expected him to deny it all so strongly. She and her sister had decided that they still did not trust him and that they would ensure that Susie was never left alone with him under any circumstances.

There are many motivations for wanting to confront an abuser or to disclose to others what happened – validation of what occurred, for factual information to complete partial memories, to make an abuser feel the impact it had on their victim, revenge, to make them suffer, to break the silence, to seek financial reparations or to warn others that there are children still at risk (Bass and Davis, 1988). They also point out, however, that 'if someone has abused you in the past, it is unlikely that person will suddenly become sensitive to your needs' (p. 135). Both Bass and Davis (1988) and Davis (1990) offer extremely helpful chapters on the issues of confrontation and disclosure.

They had not confronted their mother, having decided to talk to their father first of all. Jennifer was very emotional during the session, and most of the emotion was anger. But there was also self-doubt. Jennifer was aware that her father had left her beginning to doubt what she had heard herself saying, yet she also knew how real it had felt. She was confused.

'I feel torn apart, Laura, I don't know what to think. But I do. I heard myself speaking and I know. But I can't prove it. I don't have any clear memories, but that voice, my voice . . . .' Jennifer shivered and shook her head. She began crying. 'Could I be making it all up? But I didn't, I mean, it isn't something I had ever really thought about. It came out of the blue, it wasn't as if it was something I've been pre-occupied with. I mean, I know it happens, but I never, ever thought about it having happened to me. But could we, I, be mistaken?' Jennifer looked into Laura's eyes. 'Could I be wrong?'

Laura could sense the anguish in Jennifer's world as she asked the question of her, and of herself. She empathised with the anguish and her struggle to trust her feelings. 'It's hard to trust your own feelings?'

Jennifer went quiet. Could she be wrong? It didn't feel wrong, but it felt so hard to trust herself. Her father was saying no, and she did respect him. She thought she loved him, or at least, until recently. But he was her father. He wouldn't lie to her, would he? Would he? The more she thought about it the more confused she felt. And she could feel a headache coming on.

'I don't feel wrong, but I feel so torn. He seemed so adamant that it hadn't happened, that he had not abused me.'

'You don't feel wrong but you feel torn, and your father was so adamant . . . .' Laura had emphasised the 'so adamant' and she was unable to finish her sentence as Jennifer interrupted.

'Too adamant, he was too adamant, wouldn't even listen, or at least I didn't feel heard. My sister was good. She was so supportive but she must be wondering what to believe. I know we talked it through afterwards, and she is playing it safe with Susie, but ... oh Laura, I don't want her to stop believing me. But I can't prove anything.'

'You experienced him as too adamant, you didn't feel heard and you really don't want to feel your sister will stop believing you. And yet you are left feeling that you can't prove anything. An awful dilemma.'

Jennifer shook her head. 'Ian believes me. He was all for going to the police again, but I said no, what could I say to them? I have no memories, Laura, and oh God I don't know whether I want them or not.' She put her head in her hands and began to sob. Laura reached over to her and placed her hand on her shoulder. Jennifer turned and Laura found herself holding Jennifer in her arms.

'Oh why did all this happen? I wish I hadn't had that session now. If I hadn't heard myself speaking I wouldn't have been in this place now, would I? Oh, if I could turn the clock back. But I can't. This is where I am and I don't know what to do, I really don't.' The tears continued to flow.

The client is focused on experiencing her not knowing and the counsellor stays with this. She is not tempted to try to rescue her from the pain of not knowing by offering some positive perspective. This can be hard and testing for the counsellor, but the person-centred counsellor seeks to maintain her empathic sensitivity to what the client is experiencing and communicating.

Bass and Davis (1991) contains helpful information concerning the issues that arise for partners of survivors during their healing.

Laura could feel the jerkiness of Jennifer's breath and could sense the pain that was wracking her. She closed her eyes as she could feel her own tears welling up. She found herself staying momentarily with her own pain, which she was feeling for Jennifer as she held her. She could feel her grip tightening.

'I don't know, I just don't know.'

'Just don't know,' Laura responded and continued to hold Jennifer, whose grip had begun to relax. She felt Jennifer pulling back and so she released her. Jennifer picked up a tissue and dabbed at her eyes and blew her nose.

'I feel I want to be angry with you. All this. It wouldn't have happened if ....' Jennifer burst into tears again. 'I'm sorry, that's not fair. It isn't your fault. I know that, but I feel so angry.' She looked up. 'You do believe me, don't you?'

Laura knew that she did, although she, like Jennifer, had only heard the childhood voices speaking in the earlier session. It had felt real, and she had felt very affected by it. Laura brought herself back to Jennifer, she realised she had lost herself momentarily in her own thoughts, and she sensed that her hesitation in responding was likely to be misinterpreted. 'I believe that what you heard in that earlier session was very real. I think we are still exploring, you are still exploring, what happened then and in the past.'

Jennifer nodded instinctively and she closed her eyes as she did so, taking in a deep breath. 'I believe me, Laura, I do. I can't give you a reason, I can't prove it, but it felt so real, so real. It was me speaking, Laura, it was. And I have to know now, I have to. I have to know.' Jennifer went silent.

Laura nodded and spoke softly, 'You have to know'.

'How do I find out? I mean, I can't explore what I can't remember.' Jennifer had brought the palms of her hands together, and brought her fingers up to her lips. She parted her hands. 'I just have to go with it, don't I, and see what happens.'

Laura was aware that she was nodding in response to what Jennifer had said. She didn't add anything.

Jennifer tightened her lips. 'So I guess I have to wait and see what happens now. Maybe I'll begin to remember something.' She shivered. 'I'm scared, I'm scared of what I am going to find out. Part of me still wants to shut it away, but I know I can't. I have to know what happened.'

'Yeah, it's scary, you're scared and part of you wants to shut it all away, but another part wants to know.' Laura paused. 'I want to say that facing the unknown in ourselves takes a lot of courage. Yes, part of you wants to run away, but another part is standing with that courage wanting to face it, and probably scared witless at the same time. I just needed to say that.'

The client who is facing the unknown in themselves is heroic. Does this sound too extreme? I think not. Facing the unknown in the world outside of your skin can be scary enough, but when the unknown is within you, and you know that there are monsters lurking in that unknown, it takes a lot of courage to be prepared to face it. The real pioneers in therapy today are the clients. I learned this many years ago listening to the late Ian Gordon Brown, the co-founder of transpersonal psychology, at a conference in London. The theorists simply follow the trail that has been blazed by the clients, as it should be.

Jennifer closed her eyes and nodded. She was grateful to hear that. Yes, part of her was scared witless and wanted to run, but another part wasn't going to run but stand and face the truth. She didn't think of herself as courageous and would have found it hard to own that concept of herself without the prompt from Laura. But hearing her speak those words . . . 'Thanks for that. I appreciate it. Yes, I have the courage, I am going to come through all this.'

'You have that courage and you are going to come through it.' Laura nodded and smiled.

Jennifer held the thought of her courage for a few more moments and then became aware that her thoughts were drifting to the week ahead and knowing that she was away at another conference and couldn't make it to counselling next week. She looked at the clock, only a few minutes left.

Laura noticed the glance at the clock. 'Yes, just a few minutes left.'

'I feel I need to somehow prepare myself to be ready for anything, and it feels very shaky, I feel very shaky. I feel like I am walking into the unknown, or rather, that the unknown is walking towards me. I've got to walk towards it, Laura, whatever. I'm so glad I have you, and Ian, and Angie.' She paused. 'OK, I have to get myself together and head back home. Thanks Laura.'

The session drew to a close and Jennifer left, feeling very unsettled and yet determined to face whatever she needed to face. She was determined. She wanted to get on with her life. She had a great relationship with Ian. Her eyes moistened again as she thought about him, about how good and supportive he was being. She took in a deep breath as she got to her car and opened the door. As she got in and clicked the seat belt the thought struck her that she needed a seat belt for life, not just for driving. She knew she had people around her who supported her, but she also knew that she was alone, that this was her process, her life, her memories, her past, present and future. She gripped the steering wheel, aware that she was holding it longer than necessary and felt herself smile and her jaw tighten. She could feel her stomach churning but somehow her head felt clear, clearest it had been all evening. She had to know and she was going to know and she was going to get her past and any effect it was having on her now sorted out. She turned the key and accelerated away, the strength of her determination mirrored in the pressure she was placing on the accelerator pedal.

Supervision

Laura began by telling Malcolm how Jennifer had been to her parents and confronted her father, who had denied everything. She went on to describe how Jennifer had remembered the look on her father's face when her niece was sitting on his lap, and how it matched the image she had of his facial expression in her dreams. She described how she had used the phrase 'abuser of little girls', and was aware that it had come out of her own strong feeling, yet it had also felt very relevant and appropriate.

Malcolm sensed that Laura had her own strong feelings and wanted to offer an opportunity for her to explore them, in case they were cutting across her ability to stay within the client's frame of reference.

'Somehow when I heard myself say that it was like cutting through everything and coming down to the basics of it all, it somehow shocked me, and it shocked Jennifer and yet it was reality.'

'So how are you feeling now as you tell me this?'

Laura was aware of feeling a curious mix of anger and a sense of tenderness towards Jennifer. 'Angry comes to mind first. The bastard, and he has denied it. But I feel for Jennifer, and her family as well, as it is now coming out into the open.'

'Anger towards the bastard and feelings for Jennifer and her family.'

'Yes, I just feel so sorry for them, with what they now have to face up to and resolve in some way. What a mess. But I guess I am particularly concerned at her father's denial and the impact that is having on Jennifer.'

Malcolm couldn't help finding himself responding, 'and on you'.

'Yes. I shouldn't be surprised. I know how often the survivor is met with denial even though, what is it, only 1% of allegations of abuse turn out to be false?'

Malcolm nodded, 'Yes, and isn't it the case as well that even where there is medical evidence that abuse has taken place, when interviewed as adults up to 38% have no memory of it?'

'As high as that? Mmmm. Makes you think, the scale of it and how much remains hidden.' She shuddered. 'So, he has denied it. I know we are assuming sexual abuse occurred. Jennifer has no clear memories, not yet anyway.' Laura went quiet and thought about it. 'Yet things are going on for Jennifer. She has experienced some strange detached feelings. Like she is sort of out of her body. But I guess I have to be open to the not knowing and allow Jennifer to discover within herself what is present.'

Malcolm nodded, 'Yes, maintain that openness and that attitude of allowing,' and he added, 'and not doubt the reality of what Jennifer describes.'

The person-centred counsellor is not Sherlock Holmes or Hercule Poirot, trying to put all the pieces together and discover the truth. At best he or she has the function of enabling the client to become aware of all the pieces, but it is for the client to fit them together and draw their own conclusion. What matters is that the counsellor stays with Jennifer's thoughts and feelings without making assumptions that might distort empathy and generate incongruence. The reality for the person-centred counsellor to respond to is that of the client.

'It feels really messy. I mean, so many people are involved now. They haven't told Jennifer's mother. But they are definitely going to avoid letting her niece stay with her parents. Yet, as you say, no clear memory but a hell of a lot of indicators.'

Malcolm nodded. 'So, what is your role here?'

'To listen. Be there for Jennifer. Allow her to bring to the sessions whatever she is experiencing. Allow her to explore her own meanings attached to those experiences, and maybe develop new ones, but they must be freely her own. Be warm and supportive of her as a person. Listen to how she is experiencing things and try to keep my frame of reference out of it.' Laura smiled. 'Sounds so easy doesn't it?'

'It isn't easy. It takes a disciplined focus. Person-centred working is a hard discipline, as you know. What you have described, it is not easy.'

'No. Her father gets in the way. It's strange I don't have any really distinctive sense of him, and yet he has stirred up a strong reaction in me.'

'So he's kind of distant and yet you have a strong reaction to him.'

'Yes, and I have to put my reactions to him aside, I know that.'

'What reactions?'

Laura smiled. She knew the reactions that were present for her. 'Judge and jury. I have him guilty, don't I? I have taken sides with Jennifer.' She thought about it for a moment. 'I wonder if this is a woman-to-woman thing?'

'Woman-to-woman?' Malcolm reflected back as a question and waited.

'How might I feel if I was a man? I mean, well, you're a man so how do you react to what you have heard me say?'

'You're right, we are male and female here discussing a very painful area of human experience and yes, there may be gender-specific issues for both of us. I am aware of having a range of feelings, sadness for Jennifer as these memories seem to surface, and for her as that little girl. But I am also aware of feelings towards the father too, and wondering how he must feel whether he abused Jennifer or not. Either way, he must be damned uncomfortable.'

'I hadn't thought of that. Yes, in a sense his denial could be expected, whether he is guilty or innocent. But it makes it so hard for Jennifer.'

Gender identity can and will impact on this process. It has to be watched for. It can be obvious and it can be subtle. It can leave a counsellor or supervisor projecting feelings on to the perpetrator or the victim emerging out of their common or opposite gender identity. The attempt is to be made to avoid the risk of feelings towards the perpetrator or the victim obscuring empathy for the client. Not always easy, but always necessary.

Malcolm nodded, unsure as to where the conversation was now leading.

'It does,' he finally responded, and then added, 'I feel really bogged down with this somehow, it seems heavy, fuzzy, just hard to get a hold of somehow. Like you were saying, her father seems distant.' Malcolm was making a mental note to take his reaction to his own supervision.

'Shadowy is the word that comes to my mind, and yet I have no evidence for this, but it is a feeling that I have. I need to work at keeping my focus in Jennifer's frame of reference, I can see how easy it is to slide out of that and into my own feelings and reactions.'

'OK, do you want to explore anything else in relation to Jennifer?'

Laura thought for a moment. 'No, I think what our exploration has done for me is to give me a sense of balance, that there is a lot that is not known, and that I have to be really focused on Jennifer's experiences. I think I can find myself relating more to the whole family system, even though we have not talked about it, and empathising with each person's anguish or role in the past and the present.' Laura paused. 'What is really present for me now is this sense of really not knowing what will happen next, whether other memories will emerge and what they might be.'

Points for discussion

- Is it appropriate to counsel a client who is heavily affected by medication? At what point might it be inappropriate to continue, and who would make that decision?
- Discuss the legal implications for the counsellor of what has been disclosed.
- What are your own feelings at this point about the reality of Jennifer's accusation of her father?
- If you were the counsellor and Jennifer had no supportive network in her life, what impact might that have on your feelings and responses?
- Did Laura have to bring the focus on to Susie (Jennifer's niece), and if so, why?
- There were times when Laura shifted away from an empathic focus. Can you identify them?
- If you were jotting down thoughts, feelings, speculations at the end of Session 39, what would you be writing?
- Consider whether, when Laura introduces the topic of courage in facing the unknown, was she simply speaking to Jennifer, or might she also have been speaking to herself?
- Critically evaluate the supervision session.
- Discuss the impact of gender when working with adult survivors of child sexual abuse?

CHAPTER 7

Counselling session 42

'I've had a dream, Laura, a really bad dream.'

Laura nodded, sensing the importance of what was being said and not wanting to take anything away from Jennifer's focus. Jennifer stayed silent, and then continued.

'It was when I was away at the conference last week.'

Jennifer went silent again and Laura waited, sensing that Jennifer needed the space to disclose what she wanted at her own pace and in her own time.

'It was awful, but I know now . . . .' The words trailed off. Laura waited again.

'I had this dream, and I've had it again since the first time, but it wasn't just a dream. It felt too . . . ,' she closed her eyes, 'it felt too damn real. It was awful.'

Laura nodded. She spoke gently. 'Something about the dream was really awful.'

'I'm finding it hard to tell you about it, Laura, it seems so crazy. I can't explain it but I know what I have experienced, three times now.' Jennifer began to sob, quietly at first but gradually it became more intense. She eventually reached for a tissue, dried her eyes and looked up. 'I was abused by my father, Laura, I've seen it happen.'

'You've seen it happen?'

Jennifer nodded. 'I was kind of drifting off to sleep one night, I think I was drifting off, and I suddenly – it's hard to describe.' Jennifer swallowed and went silent.

'Take your time.'

'You might think I'm mad, but I saw it happening, Laura, I saw it happening. And I can still see it now.'

'I don't think you are mad, Jennifer, but I sense how difficult it is to share this dream, this memory with me.'

Jennifer smiled. 'Thanks for that. Yes. It is difficult. Seemed so easy as I was driving over, but now it all seems a bit crazy. But I know it happened.'

'You know it happened.'

Jennifer took a deep breath. 'I was about 10 or 11 I think, not sure, and I could see myself lying on the bed.' Her voice became more difficult to hear as she continued. 'My father was lying on top of me.'

Laura nodded and reached out to take Jennifer's hand. Jennifer took it and gripped it tightly. 'He was fucking me.' Jennifer could feel the waves of emotion hit her and she burst into tears again. She struggled to continue between the sobs and the tears. 'He was fucking me. I could see his arse moving up and down, pushing down into me. He was inside me. I couldn't feel it in the dream. I seemed to be out of my body, looking at what was happening. Is that possible?'

Laura nodded, not wanting to get into a technical discussion, but wanting to acknowledge the reality of what Jennifer was describing.

'I just watched. He was talking to me all the time, telling me how special I was, and how much my mother didn't understand him, that I was his little girl and he kept saying to me, "you are enjoying this, aren't you, you're enjoying this". I wasn't but I remember feeling so afraid. And when he finished and got up and left the room I kind of fell back into my body. Oh God the pain. I felt torn apart, as if I'd been ripped in two. I felt that in the dream, I felt myself coming back into my body and feeling waves of pain.' Jennifer had moved forward in the chair and was clutching her knees, and rocking slightly. 'It was awful, and it's so vivid, so real, so with me.' The tears flowed down her cheeks as she continued to rock silently back and forth.

'So much pain. So much pain.'

Jennifer nodded. 'The memory is with me now. It isn't just something in a dream any more. And on one of the times when I had the dream, it was different, there was a different-coloured duvet. It must have happened more than once.' Jennifer shivered. 'I'm suddenly feeling very cold, I need to go and sit with my back to the radiator.' She got up and sat on the floor on a cushion against the radiator.

'You can now remember the experience, it isn't just a dream. And it happened more than once. It isn't just a dream.'

Jennifer shook her head. 'No.' She stared ahead of her for a while and Laura sat and waited. Eventually Laura quietly said, 'No need to say anything more unless you want to.'

Jennifer heard Laura's voice but she could sense that it had become distant somehow. Everything seemed distant. She curled up more tightly. 'I couldn't stop him, Laura, I couldn't stop him.'

'I hear you saying that you couldn't stop him, you were only a 10-year-old girl, Jennifer, you were only a 10-year-old girl.'

The victim of child sexual abuse can blame themselves, feeling they should have been able to stop it happening, questioning whether they had encouraged it, made it happen. The encouragement by the perpetrator that the victim is enjoying it, and is special because they have been chosen to experience it, is not unusual. What Laura is trying to hold Jennifer on is the fact that she was only a 10-year-old girl, and therefore basically powerless against her father. The unvoiced implication is that she was not to blame, that the responsibility lies with her father. It may take time for the client to reach this awareness for themselves.

'Yes, I was only a 10-year-old girl, and I can't help feeling responsible, and I know you are right, but my feelings tell me I must have encouraged it, I must have enjoyed it. But I know I didn't.' Jennifer tucked her head into her arms and stayed curled up. ' I should feel angry, Laura, I should hate him, but I can't reach those feelings. I just feel ... I mean, I just feel numb. It's like watching a film only then you realise you are in it. I just feel so much hurt.' With that Jennifer broke down in tears again.

Laura spoke softly and slowly, describing what she had heard, allowing Jennifer to experience her inner world having been listened to, heard and validated. 'You know you were not responsible but you are experiencing feelings that you must have been. You feel you should hate him, but you feel numb towards him, and you feel so much hurt in yourself.'

'Oh God, what am I going to do? I don't know how to cope with it all.'

'Feels hard to see how to cope?'

'Yes, but people do, I know they do. Oh, and the drinking's gone up again. My doctor switched me to 2 mg tablets and I had reduced down, but now I'm drinking again in the evenings.'

'Taking the pain away, yeah?' Laura spoke softly.

'Yes. It helps, but it isn't the answer. What do I do?' Jennifer got up. 'I'm feeling stiff.' She stretched and returned to her chair.

This is a clear case of where the person-centred counsellor trusts the client's process. The memories have surfaced at this time, they have not been forced to the surface, and Laura knows that she must trust Jennifer to make the choices she needs to make in order to cope with the memories that are now so very present for her.

'What do you feel you need to do, Jennifer?'

'I can't get rid of the memories, and I can't keep using alcohol to cope with them. I have to find the strength within me to carry these memories.' Jennifer lapsed into silence. 'Oh God, I feel so small, I feel so terrified.'

'Small and terrified?'

'I can feel myself lying in my bed, all curled up. I'm crying into the pillow. I hurt so much. I ache. The pain. Oh God.' Tears flowed once more and the sobs got louder and heavier.

Laura moved closer. Jennifer had her head in her hands and was rocking in the chair. She remained like that for some minutes, sobbing continuously and every now and then uttering strangled sounds from her throat of pain and anguish. Laura had noted the time and was not concerned as to whether Jennifer was going to be able to bring herself back out in order to drive home, at least not yet. She simply spoke quietly every now and then, 'I'm here for you, Jennifer, I'm here for you.'

Time passed, the tears continued to flow, the pain ... the pain persisted. But it was no longer a remembering of the physical pain, it was increasingly a pain that tore at the very soul of her being, a dirty, used, abused, unclean pain. Heavy, dark, oppressive, but most of all it had a feel of filth about it that would not go away. Somewhere in the midst of the darkness Jennifer could sense Laura's continued presence. It felt so lonely where she was but it felt so good to have someone there, someone she could trust, that she knew wouldn't abandon her. It was something to hang on to. Her head was throbbing and her eyes felt red raw. She felt sick but it was more of a burning feeling that rose up in her chest and throat. She screwed her eyes up as she felt another wave of burning pain, it seemed to extend from her crotch up through her body, like red hot metal had been thrust up into her body. She began to tremble, her body shaking of its own volition. She could do nothing to stop it. Then she suddenly felt herself going cold, and sweating. 'I suddenly feel so cold.' Laura took Jennifer's coat down and wrapped it around her shoulders. 'Thanks.' She continued to tremble and shake. 'It's like my body is not mine anymore,' she stuttered, and she tried to brace herself and stop the trembling, but it would not stop. 'Oh God, I-I've never felt anything like this before.'

'Your body is reacting to everything, Jennifer, a kind of release.' Laura wanted to offer her some reassurance. 'Your body is releasing some of the trauma.'

Memories seem to be stored not just in the brain, but in the body as well. Jennifer's body is reliving the experience, it is not just a memory of the past. This reliving will help her to integrate the experience into her awareness and will reduce the fragmentation and the tension in the body. Sometimes painful and distressing physical symptoms can emerge out of this remembering by the body, causing added anxiety and discomfort for the client. 'Memories are stored in our bodies and it is possible to re-experience the terror of the abuse. Your body may clutch tight, or you may feel the screams you could not scream as a child. Or you may feel that you are suffocating and cannot breathe' (Bass and Davis, 1988, p. 75). See also Sanderson (1995) and Kepner (1995).

The body, like the emotions and the mind, needs to feel the presence of empathy, unconditional warmth and authenticity in the therapist. Often reassuring physical contact can convey this. But it should be spontaneous and flow from a genuine empathic sensitivity to the need of the client, and not the need of the therapist.

Jennifer nodded and realised that she was gritting her teeth. The tension she was feeling, all her muscles were tensed. She felt an enormous wave of emotion, anger, rage, fury. 'You fucking, fucking bastard. I hate you. You did this to me.' Jennifer was still shaking, her knuckles were white. She was shaking her head from side to side. She looked up at Laura. 'He's going to know what he did to me, what I am experiencing. But not yet. I'm still remembering, I want him to hear it all.' She spat the words out with venom. As she said this Jennifer could feel the shaking begin to reduce and the tension ease. 'How much more of this have I got to go through?'

'I don't know, Jennifer, I don't know how much there is to remember.' She felt so much, but she couldn't put it into words. Yes, she felt compassion for Jennifer, and she felt pain for her, and she felt angry, and sad that this happened, and how damaging and painful it was. And how it reached into everything about the person who was the target of child sexual abuse. 'I feel so much for you, Jennifer.'

Jennifer could feel a strength inside herself, coming from somewhere deep. 'I'm going to come through this, Laura, I'm going to survive this.' The clock had caught her eye and Laura had noticed it.

'You're going to survive, Jennifer, you're going to survive.' She spoke slowly, speaking directly to the part of Jennifer that was carrying her determination to come through this experience. She didn't mention the time, it would have cut across the moment, and she knew Jennifer had noticed it. She wanted to help Jennifer hold her focus on her determination.

'Yes.' There was suddenly a very unfeeling tone to Jennifer's voice. 'Yes.' She nodded. To Laura she looked rather distant, as if she was looking towards a distant horizon.

'You look as though you are looking a long way into the, I'm not sure, future, past, somewhere distant.'

'I feel different. I somehow feel focused. And I know I am wondering what else I'm going to remember, but I've started and there's no going back now. I want to know what happened to me. But I want to know from my experience. It's my memory, my life. I've experienced, relived something of what happened, and I have come through it. I take comfort from that. ' She closed her eyes as she felt the flow of tears and the upsurge of emotion. She struggled to speak as the tears continued. 'It was my childhood and it was my body . . . .' Her voice trailed off. 'Why?' She shook her head. 'Will I ever know?' She shook her head again. 'Don't answer that. It's getting close to time for me to go. It was an awful session but I feel somehow better for it though I also feel like I've been put through a mangle.'

'You have re-experienced so much and it has left me feeling so much respect for your courage, Jennifer. I cannot begin to imagine the pain you're are going through, it is not in my experience, but I can be touched, deeply, by the effect it is having on you, and what it feels like being close to you in this awful experience. I want to be here for you and help you find your way through this.' Laura wanted to convey in words her warmth towards Jennifer, the respect that she felt for her and commitment to the therapeutic relationship. She was deeply moved. As she finished speaking, Jennifer turned and gave her a hug. They held the embrace for some while.

The core conditions are communicated physically.

The session drew to a close and Jennifer left. Before leaving, Laura told her that if she needed to call before the next session that was OK, and she reminded her of when she was available to take calls. Jennifer appreciated that. It did feel lonely and yet she knew she wasn't alone. She had Ian, and her sister. But she also appreciated that Laura did not have an agenda, wasn't one of the family, but was someone who had this wonderful ability to just let her be how she needed to be, and to stay with her. And she was so grateful for that.

Laura was very aware of her own tiredness when Jennifer had left. It had been an emotionally draining session, so intense, so concentrated. She felt she had been trying to give out so much of herself in being present for and with Jennifer. It made her aware of how often people do not appreciate the emotional cost of being a therapist. But it was what she wanted to do. There were people out there, like Jennifer, who were deeply wounded by traumatic experiences, and she wanted to help them, and help the healing process. It was not easy, it was never easy, and at times it felt like she was standing inside her client's experiencing. She was grateful for that for she knew that if she was to be effective she had to be affected. She had to join her clients and stand beside them in their suffering.

A memory of a workshop she had attended came to mind, about working with people traumatised by war, by some of the most horrific experiences that she could imagine, some of which had made her go cold at the thought. I only have myself to offer to my clients, she thought, and that is what they need – a person – a human being, striving to gain an appreciation of their inner world of horror and pain, or whatever else is present for them. They need someone to relate to them, to reach out to them, to touch and be touched by them. She knew she had been touched by Jennifer that evening, and she hoped that in the midst of all the pain and anguish Jennifer had also felt touched by her presence as a companion, as a woman, as a person, as a human being prepared to sit with her.

Counselling session 43

Jennifer had phoned the day before the appointment to cancel. She was suffering from an infection and it had wiped her out. She said that with the infection – urinary tract – she had found herself really not thinking or feeling much about anything. That her body and her mind seemed to have gone numb. She just felt as though she didn't care about anything, and just took each moment as it came. She was feeling the effects of the antibiotics and was spending most of the time asleep. They set up the next appointment for the following week.

Counselling session 44

Jennifer began by apologising for cancelling and went on to describe how she had been during the week. She said that, in fact, she felt it had been timely for her, that things had become intense and that the week had given her a different perspective somehow. She had wondered if the infection had somehow been linked to what she was remembering and had decided to accept that possibility. She spoke of feeling a lot calmer and not sure whether that was still the effects of the infection and the treatment, or whether she had actually come to terms with things a little more. She said that as the week went on she had felt more able to reflect on things. She felt the anger was still there but that it had eased.

Over the weekend Jennifer said that she had spoken to her sister and that, given the clarity of what she had experienced in the dreams and the flashbacks, she felt she needed to speak to her father again, but that she wanted to wait a little longer. She felt she wanted more awareness of what had happened. She explored why she felt that way, wanting to check out that she really was genuinely OK with that.

Laura sensed that Jennifer was doing a lot of reflecting on the situation during the session and she agreed that she did not feel in a place in herself that week to really re-engage with her memories. Rather, she felt she needed time to just be and to talk things through and acknowledge her current position and attitude.

'For better or worse, at last it has begun to come to the surface and I can now learn to deal with it. It's not being left unprocessed. I really appreciate the way you are helping me slowly re-integrate my past. It feels unhurried, unpressured.'

Laura acknowledged this and the session moved on.

'One thing that I am conscious of and it is now troubling me because I am associating it with being abused. I have always been very conscious of wanting to be clean, I remember how I used to shower and bath a lot. I never really thought much about it, it was just what I did. But I suppose I have been a bit more self-aware lately and I am aware of feeling sort of, I don't know, anxious is too strong a word, but when I go to shower or have a bath there is a kind of edge to what is going on for me. Feels like I am sort of driven to wash, and, well, it was Ian who commented on it as well. I kind of get the feeling that I can't get myself clean, you know? Silly really, but I keep coming back to how dirty I have felt when I have remembered what happened and I, oh I don't know, but I guess I'm concerned I'm getting a bit obsessive.' Jennifer smiled weakly as she finished.

Obsessive and compulsive disorders can and do arise as symptoms of traumatic experiences such as child sexual abuse. Often they are treated cognitively but if the underlying trauma is not addressed (and it may be unknown to the client and therefore not emerge within the therapy) such treatment is unlikely to be lasting. It may bring temporary relief from the behaviours but the underlying traumatised condition remains unaffected. It's presence, even though unknown to the client, can stimulate the return of the obsessive and compulsive behaviours or they may return as the traumatised experiences emerge into awareness.

Laura could hear an edge of concern in Jennifer's voice, and the smile didn't seem very authentic. 'So, that sense of feeling dirty and of never really being able to get clean. Worried about it becoming obsessive. I hear your concern, Jennifer.'

'Well, it hadn't really struck me until last week. I guess I did spend a lot of time washing but then, well, I was running a temperature. But it somehow felt more than that.'

'Felt more than just a response to running a temperature.'

'Yes, and yet I don't want to go and obsess about it, you know? I mean, that's all I need, some obsessive behaviour. But I do spend a lot of time washing myself, and particularly between my legs and my upper thighs.' Jennifer thought for a moment. 'More than any other part of my body, and I noticed a couple of times that I really needed to kind of make myself stop. One time Ian called out because I had been in the shower so long. That was what unsettled me. Made me feel really anxious, as though I had to hurry up but I needed more time, but that was ridiculous I had already been in the shower washing myself for ages. Could I be obsessing, Laura?'

' "Obsessing" is quite a powerful word, can be an unsettling label for a behaviour. It troubles you and my sense is that you are very uneasy about the time you are spending washing.'

'I am uneasy and I don't want it to get out of control. I mean, obsessions are like addictions, aren't they, and I'm worried, you know, with my history, well, I mean, I could develop a problem.'

Whilst hearing Jennifer's unease, Laura was aware of wondering what she might want to do about it. 'It seems you are more aware of the possibility of it getting out of control and want to be sure of being in control?'

'Yes, but I really don't want to think about it, you know, I want to just be normal and I'm kind of questioning how normal I am.' Jennifer thought for a moment. Talking about this was leaving her more anxious about it.

A client can experience increased anxiety and interpret this as meaning that the counselling is making them more anxious and is therefore unhelpful. In extreme cases a client may withdraw from the counsellor for this reason. What is actually occuring is that the client is simply becoming more aware of the level of anxiety that they have, in other words, becoming more sensitive to the degree of incongruence that is present within them. Jennifer has a concept of normal, no doubt an introject from other people, and her experience of herself does not match this. And neither match her genuine potential as a person which lies obscured behind the introjects and her current experience of herself. She experiences incongruence manifested through an anxiety state.

'It is making me anxious. I need to watch myself. I need to take it a little more easy.' Jennifer stopped again and was aware that she could feel this weird sense of dirtiness creeping up on her.

'You want to feel normal and the washing doesn't feel normal. It makes you anxious and I am aware that you look troubled, Jennifer.' Laura had noticed the frown appear on Jennifer's face.

Jennifer took in a breath and opened her mouth to speak, but closed it again. It was hard to explain. 'I feel kind of dirty, soiled, somehow "secondhand".' As she said this she felt a rush of emotion that took her by surprise. 'I feel used, or at least, part of me does.'

'A part of you feels used?'

'And it's a part of me that's dirty, that doesn't care about how I look, how I look after myself.'

'A part of you that doesn't care, that's dirty ....'

Jennifer cut in. 'Yes, yes, and I live that out. I can be quite "don't care" at times, yet then this washing part of me, that doesn't fit, because that bit does care, it wants me clean but ....' Jennifer went quiet and looked a little shocked.

'You look as though you were about to say something but it shocked you.'

'I could hear the words "but doesn't think you will ever be clean" coming to mind, and that's really painful.' As she ended her sentence Jennifer's eyes moistened. 'Never be clean. No, no, I can get clean, I must get clean, I must.'

Laura noticed that Jennifer's voice had changed, a little more high-pitched. She sensed a shift and felt that Jennifer might have connected strongly to this part of her that had to get clean. 'Jennifer must get clean,' she responded softly.

'Yes, I must, I must. But I can't, I can't wash it away. I'm dirty, I'm a dirty little girl and I can't get clean. I can't but I must.'

As Jennifer sat there she began to twitch and to rub her hands together. She began to rub her thighs with her hands and then began to rub herself between the legs. 'Must get clean. Can't get clean. Always happens again. Can never get clean. Can never get clean.'

'Never get clean?' Laura responded with a questioning tone.

'But I have to. I have to. I have to ....' Jennifer stopped speaking and burst into tears, sobbing loudly.

Laura could feel a tremendous urge to say something but she knew it was not a reflection of what Jennifer was saying, yet it seemed that it was powerfully present. She didn't feel she had time to debate the issue with herself, she felt she needed to trust her instinct. 'You feel that you have to get clean, but maybe you don't have to.'

'Don't have to, don't have to. I do have to. I have to be clean. He likes me to be clean.'

Laura was shocked by the response, and Jennifer's voice had changed, sounded much younger. She had thought that the part of her needing to be clean was Jennifer as an older child, now it seemed she had slipped back into a much younger age.

'He likes you to be clean.'

'Yes, he baths me, and he washes me. He likes me to be clean.'

'Who baths you?'

'Daddy. He baths me because I am special. I like feeling special.' Jennifer's expression changed. 'But I don't like it when it hurts.'

'When it hurts?

'No, I don't like it then.'

'You don't like it when it hurts.' Laura kept her responses simple and softly spoken.

'No.' Her face brightened again, 'But I like being special.'

Jennifer has switched into a dissociated state, probably her 4-year-old self but it could be her 7-year-old state. Or maybe some curious combination of both. Either way, the switch was sudden, and so is the switch back into her usual awareness.

Jennifer's facial expression changed again. 'Oh God, Laura, what was that about? I could hear myself speaking and I felt very young again, I think like it was that time back when I was about four years old. That wasn't the part of me that was talking about feeling dirty, that was older, when I was 10 or so, when he was, when he was – what do I call it, Laura? I mean, when he was abusing me isn't how I want to say it, when he was fucking me. Shit.' Jennifer closed her eyes. 'OK.' She opened her eyes again. 'Stuff was going on when I was really young and when I was a little older. I have images from when I was older, but no images from when I was younger, only hearing myself speaking about it. Somehow I only seem to connect with that here, only seem to be able to talk about it. I can only imagine what he was doing when he was bathing me.'

'Yes, the flashbacks and memories are from later. You have no memories, other than kneeling at the window, of when you were younger. But you are hearing the voice of yourself as that very young child, at both four and seven.' Laura realised she had taken the focus away from where Jennifer had reached in what she had been saying. She brought it back, 'And you are left only with your imagination as to what he was doing when he was bathing you.'

'Yes.' Jennifer went quiet. She could only imagine, but she had no images, just thoughts, and the feelings of revulsion that came with them. Had he tried to rape her? Rape. She had consistently talked about how he had fucked her, but it wasn't that, was it, it was rape. 'He raped me, didn't he, this isn't about fucking, this was rape. I've only just thought about it in those terms. It leaves me feeling different. I was powerless. It wasn't my fault. I didn't asked to be raped. I couldn't say no. And earlier, I didn't understand what was happening, I couldn't have understood. Four years old and he starts touching me, playing with me, probably trying to get inside me. Oh God.'

'Yes, it was rape, and you were powerless, you didn't ask for it to happen, you couldn't say no, you wouldn't have understood when you were four.'

'And by the time I was seven he had already convinced me that it was what special girls did, got.' She closed her eyes. 'Oh shit, shit, shit, what a mess. And . . . this washing stuff, oh God that's a Pandora's box as well. Wanting to be clean, not thinking I can ever get clean, believing I am dirty.' Jennifer could feel herself suddenly becoming very tired, and she tried to stifle a yawn without much success. 'I feel so drained.' She sipped some water. 'I think I have done enough for this evening. I've got to get control of this needing to be clean issue, and this other "don't care" attitude.' She stopped for a moment, a sudden realisation had struck her. 'I wonder if the drinking is linked to "don't care"?'

Up to this point we have been referring to the notion of 'dissociated parts'. The 'don't care' part of Jennifer is something else and may well be regarded as a 'drinking configuration' (Bryant-Jefferies, 2001, 2003), a 'configuration of self' (Mearns, 1988, 1999, 2000) that in this example has adopted alcohol use as one of its distinguishing behaviours. The concept of configurations is not to be thought of as being on some kind of continuum with Dissociative Identity Disorder (DID). Both Mearns (2000) and Warner (2000) are clear on this. Mearns writes, 'a "configuration" is a hypothetical construct denoting a coherent pattern of feelings, thoughts and preferred behavioural responses symbolised or pre-symbolised by the person as reflective of a dimension of existence within the Self' (p. 102). He goes on to make the point that 'in considering Self in regard to "configurations", we are embracing "normal" dimensions of personality integration' (p. 108). In contrast, dissociative parts develop in response to extreme traumatic experiencing in childhood. They have greater individual identity and a more profound separateness from each other.

'The idea that your drinking is associated with the "don't care" you?'
'That makes sense somehow, though I need to think about it more.' Jennifer yawned again. 'Sorry, I think I've pretty much exhausted myself this evening. Probably still recovering from last week.'
The session drew to a close, Jennifer confirmed that she felt OK to drive home.
Laura reflected on the session and her sense that she had encountered some of Jennifer's configurations of self. There was something associated with her don't care attitude and feeling dirty, which may be linked to her alcohol use; then there might be a sense of self that she associated with being special with her father when she was so very young; and then that part of her that was urging her to get clean which seemed to be a reaction to the part of her that felt dirty, used and, what was it she had said, oh yes, feeling secondhand. So much to hold and to be attentive to. And Laura knew, as well, that they had only really just begun unravelling what had happened in the past and the impact it had had on Jennifer's structure of self.

Counselling session 45

'I've remembered more, Laura, I've been experiencing more flashbacks. Some have been with me lying there with him on top of me, touching me, inside me, raping me.' Jennifer's voice seemed somehow devoid of all emotion. And yet the atmosphere in the room was electric.

Laura stayed with what Jennifer had said and reflected it back. 'Remembering him on top of you, touching you, inside you, raping you.' Laura was aware that she was feeling emotion as she spoke, a huge longing to reach out and hold Jennifer, and yet she held back, knowing that to act on this impulse would perhaps direct Jennifer away from what she may now want to disclose.

'Inside me.' Jennifer shivered and Laura could feel the emptiness in her own stomach, a cold emptiness that left her feeling sick. She nodded and responded, keeping her empathic focus on what Jennifer was saying.

'Inside you.'

Jennifer closed her eyes. As she had begun speaking the experience had somehow grown closer once more. She seemed to be able to distance herself from it most of the time, but it had once again become all too real. She pulled herself away from it, deliberately, and her thoughts went back to Friday evening.

'I was lying in bed on Friday evening, I had gone up early and had been reading, waiting for Ian who was watching the end of some football on TV. I felt drowsy and put the book aside. I heard the TV go off and I must have drifted in that moment. I feel a numbness now as I recall it.' Jennifer went silent.

'So you were waiting for Ian and felt drowsy, and recalling it now is leaving you feeling numb.'

'I was lying there and then suddenly I wasn't, at least I was but I wasn't. I felt this tremendous pressure inside my head and a kind of buzzing sound, and I felt so heavy, so heavy. I feel heavy now as I talk about it.'

'You're feeling heavy.'

Jennifer stayed silent. She felt hesitant at saying what happened next although she felt Laura would understand. But it felt difficult to put into words even though she had recalled the experience a number of times now, but on this occasion it had been different, horribly different.

'You know how I have said before that I could recall being above my body looking down, watching what he was doing to me?'

Laura nodded, 'Yes, I remember.'

'Well, it happened again on Friday. And again on Saturday when Ian and I made love, and I think I may have felt that before in the past with other men, but I'm not sure. But it is Friday that shocked me, Laura, really shocked me.' Jennifer lapsed into silence again.

Laura respected Jennifer's need for silence and quietly said, after about half a minute, 'What happened Friday really shocked you.'

Jennifer nodded but her head stayed down. She looked up, looking deep into Laura's eyes as she did so. It was a look that was so full of hurt and pain that Laura knew her facial expression must have reacted. She voiced her reaction. 'You look so full of hurt and pain, Jennifer.'

Jennifer closed her eyes and she could feel them watering. She opened them and tears trickled down both cheeks. 'It wasn't what he was doing, I was up above it all, looking down, I could see him and hear him grunting as he thrusted into me. But it was not him that I saw.' Jennifer could feel the goose bumps breaking out all over her body. 'She was in the doorway.'

Laura's first thought was to Jennifer's sister, but she brought herself back from this to simply reflect back questioningly, inviting further disclosure. 'She was in the doorway?'

Jennifer nodded. 'She was watching but saying nothing, just stood there, and then I saw her turn and walk away.' Again she looked deeply into Laura's eyes. 'She turned and walked away. She did nothing, nothing.' At this point Jennifer broke down in tears, really broke down. It was terrible to witness – the pain, the hurt, the wails that emerged from her throat. Laura instinctively reached over and held her hand, both her hands. She closed her own eyes and allowed her own feelings to be present. She took a deep breath and brought herself back to focus on Jennifer who was continuing to cry with the same intensity.

Through the tears and her struggle to breathe Jennifer spoke, the words coming out between sharp intakes of breath. 'She-watched-and-she-walked-away.'

This wasn't her sister, Laura realised, oh no, there was only one other person it could be. She instinctively felt herself squeezing Jennifer's hands tighter. She did not know what to say, so she just continued to hold Jennifer's hands.

Out-of-body experiences can occur in moments of extreme trauma and shock. If they are a feature of a person's dissociated process then they may be left with a tendency to enter this state. This can be triggered in response to events and experiences later in life which, whilst they may not carry the traumatic intensity of the causative experiences, are likely to have a similarity or resonance to that original event and the feelings that were intensely aroused at the time. For instance, a later experience of intense fear, powerlessness, anxiety and pain could trigger the person into not only an associated state but also an out-of-body state. Whilst some argue it is all a brain-centred fantasy experience, the reality can be that the person sees things that they simply could not have seen from where they were physically positioned. What happened to Jennifer is a case of this. She has seen someone in the doorway who she would not otherwise have been aware of.

Bass and Davis refer to this process as 'splitting', suggesting that in its milder form the individual flees to a mental level to get away from feelings and bodily experience, but that in extreme cases the person actually leaves the body, a 'feat', they describe, 'as something yogis work decades to achieve', but which 'comes naturally to children during severe trauma' (Bass and Davis, 1988, pp. 209–10). It leaves the person with a predisposition to going 'out-of-body', it can become like an instinctive method of escape, a survival mechanism, as if a doorway has been found and opened allowing consciousness in some way to escape from fearful situations. Going out-of-body can be a conscious choice, or it can be an unconscious, instinctively driven reaction.

'She did nothing, nothing. But she can't have forgotten.' Jennifer looked at Laura. 'She knows. She knows.'

Laura stayed with what Jennifer was saying. 'She did nothing but she knows.'

'I could see her face quite clearly. It was strange, seeing her from above. She was looking at me, at him, but she couldn't have known that I was seeing her. Her face looked,' Jennifer hesitated, 'she looked empty, pale, almost lifeless. I'd never seen her look like that. Like all the colour had drained out of her face. But she did nothing, that's what hurts so much, she did nothing. She left him with me.' Jennifer closed her eyes again as the sick feeling returned and she felt her throat dry out. She took a few sips of water and a few deep breaths. 'How could she do nothing?'

'That's what really hurts – how could she do nothing?'

'I feel hot, cold, sick, but most of all I feel betrayed.'

'Betrayed?' Laura reflected but in a way that invited further comment.

'She was supposed to protect me, that's what mothers do, don't they? She was supposed to protect me, but she just watched and turned away. She left me to him.' Jennifer could feel anxiety building up inside her. 'I don't understand, I feel confused. My head, I feel, oh I feel like I could pass out.' She could feel a cold sweat breaking out over her face.

Laura had noticed the colour draining out of Jennifer's face just before she ended her sentence, and caught her in her arms as her head flopped forward. She eased her back into the chair and as she did so Jennifer opened her eyes. 'I feel so weak.' She could feel her head swimming and the temptation to just droop back into a faint was very present. 'I need to lower my head, get the blood back.' Jennifer dropped her head down and held it in her hands. Gradually she felt her strength returning, and the cold sweat was retreating. She took a deep breath as she lifted her head and reached for the water.

'Phew, I really reacted to that.' Her hand was trembling as she reached over for the glass.

'It's really shaken you,' Laura replied, noticing how shaky Jennifer looked.

'I seem to be feeling more about my mother than my father somehow. As though I am blanking him out, but I can't blank her out. I just feel so incredibly fragile.'

'Yeah, so very, very fragile,' Laura responded, letting Jennifer know that she had heard and appreciated what she was saying to her.

Jennifer sat for a moment, she could feel herself trembling, and not just physically. She just felt so disturbed by it all. It felt like she was in her body but somehow slightly out of herself, like she had been jarred loose in some strange way.

'I feel like I'm on the edge of myself.'

Laura felt herself frown as she struggled to appreciate what Jennifer meant by this, and realised she was not sure. 'On the edge of yourself?'

The counsellor responds empathically with a tone of questioning in order to encourage more. The temptation can be to own the fact of struggling to understand, and this could appear reasonable, but it would run the risk of taking the client's focus from what she is experiencing to concerns as to the counsellor's difficulty. Whilst it may be an expression of counsellor's authenticity, the need for maintaining empathy overrides this.

Jennifer just nodded. Hearing that phrase repeated back to her somehow made a strong impression. She could feel a reaction around her solar plexus. It felt very wobbly. She could feel a kind of tickly sensation in her arms and it seemed as though her stomach was being gently squeezed. It didn't feel at all pleasant. She continued to sit with this sensation. She didn't feel any urge to speak. It was like being in suspended animation. She didn't know how much time had passed but she heard Laura say, 'I'm here for you.' She felt herself nod slightly but she did not respond in any other way. The sensations in her body were very present, and she felt like they were holding her attention and her focus. She remembered again how it had felt to find herself out of her body. Funnily enough, she had felt quite calm about it, it hadn't been that in itself that had been disturbing. It had been seeing her mother. As that image came back to her she felt the other calmer sensations fade. She was aware that she was shaking her head slightly from side to side. What she was experiencing was utter disbelief. How could she? How could she? She was aware that water was building up in her eyes and she felt a tear trickle down her left cheek.

Laura had noticed the tear but chose to say nothing. She knew that something was happening for Jennifer, that she needed to be there and remain attentive. She did say, 'I don't know what you are experiencing but I am here for you if you want to share it.' She was struck by a sense of how lonely it must have been for Jennifer to carry her experiences in childhood. She realised she was assuming that there had been no one to talk to about them, but that was so often the case. The secret was carried and dissociated, too painful to hold in everyday awareness. In a way, it was a blessing that the psychological system could work like that, it brought some relief, but it was always at a cost when memories re-emerged.

Jennifer was still very much in her own experiencing and yet she was also aware that she was feeling an appreciation that she was not on her own, that Laura was there even though they were not talking about it. Having a presence, someone who cared, someone who, well, was just there, somehow made a huge difference. She wasn't alone with it as she sat there. Somehow she felt a little stronger knowing that Laura was there, quietly sitting, a warm and consistent presence that she could trust. As this feeling struck her she could feel the tears well up more strongly and her throat dried. She could feel the sentence forming in her mind, 'I wish Laura had been there, she wouldn't have looked and turned away.' She didn't voice it, the tears and the emotions overtook her.

Without realising what was happening for Jennifer, Laura was aware of a sudden rush of motherly feeling for her, a real sense of wanting to protect her from everything. She felt a little buzzy in her head as she experienced this and she just knew she had to reach out and hold her, she couldn't explain why, but she just had to, like she was being commanded to. She got out of the chair, went across and took Jennifer in her arms. The reaction from Jennifer was instant. The distress poured out of her and minutes passed with Laura holding Jennifer, who was gently rocking whilst crying and sobbing.

For Jennifer, Laura's moving over to hold her had caught her in the exact moment that she had wished Laura had been there for her as a child. The flood of feelings that hit her in that moment just engulfed her. Not just feelings of hurt, but also a real yearning, a tremendous wanting to be held, to be held in a way that made her feel heard and loved and cared for. The need to be loved, she realised how much she needed to be loved, and she clung on to Laura like she never wanted to let her go – ever.

Sometimes the therapist will connect with the client at some deep level that will trigger a behaviour in the counsellor that they may, or may not, make sense of, but which turns out to be right. Rogers wrote of how when he was closest to his 'inner, intuitive self', that whatever he did 'seemed to be full of healing'. He said that he could not force the experience but that when he could be close to the transcendental core of himself, he might 'behave in strange and impulsive ways in the relationship, ways which I cannot justify rationally, which have nothing to do with my thought processes. But these strange behaviours seem to be *right*, in some odd way; it seems that my inner spirit has reached out and touched the inner spirit of the other. Our relationship transcends itself and becomes part of something larger. Profound growth and healing and energy are present' (Rogers, 1980, p. 129).

The fact of the timing of Laura's response coinciding with Jennifer's unvoiced felt need could be seen to be indicative of a deeper connectivity between them in that moment, inducing an action in Laura that had the quality of 'rightness' alluded to by Rogers.

As time passed, Jennifer began to experience an easing of the feelings, and she relaxed her grip on Laura. 'Thank you.' She took a deep breath. 'Thank you.'

Laura smiled and also released her hold on Jennifer, 'Shall I stay here beside you?'

'Yes please. Your being close feels very important at the moment.'

Laura moved her chair next to Jennifer's and she sat next to her with her arm around her.

Jennifer closed her eyes for a moment. 'Feels good.'

'Mmmm?'

'Feels good. I didn't realise until now how much I needed to be held, to be loved. You reached out to me when I most needed it and wham, I was hit by a tidal wave of feelings. And it was good, it was good. I needed it.' She took another deep breath, 'I needed it.'

Laura responded with empathy for what Jennifer was telling her. 'You hadn't realised just how much you needed to feel loved, just how much you needed to be held . . . .' She didn't get a chance to finish before Jennifer responded.

'No idea, it seemed to come from somewhere very deep inside me, very, very deep. I felt very small and the feelings were so big.' Jennifer paused for a moment, and continued. 'It feels good, I somehow feel good. I somehow feel a bit stronger, and that seems to be linked to you being here, being close, listening, caring. You didn't need to say anything, but you were there. That's what I didn't get. I feel like I've released something. Not that I think I've released everything, but it feels important, very, very important. I somehow feel a little calmer now.' She paused again and smiled. 'And you don't need to repeat that all back to me, I know you've heard me.'

They looked at each other and something shifted in their relationship. Something that was hard for either of them to define and yet there was a knowing that somehow everything was OK.

Laura responded to the experience. 'I have a tremendous sense that all is and will be OK, but I'm not sure what it is about and I am curious if that has any meaning for you.'

What Laura is experiencing and voicing has emerged out of her empathic connection and sense of relatedness with Jennifer. It is an appropriate voicing of congruent experiencing because of this.

Jennifer smiled. 'That's how it seems to me. I feel like I know what happened in the past. OK, I haven't all the details, but I know that I was sexually abused by my father and that my mother was aware. That is my reality and I must live with it. But as I say that, I am also feeling a warm calm, a kind of acceptance somehow of that was how it is and I must get on with life. And what I am experiencing most is a sense that "I am OK".' Jennifer spoke the words without any undue emphasis on any of them.

Laura trusted her sense of needing to respond to those last three words, 'I am OK', and reflected them back but more slowly than Jennifer had, although again avoiding undue emphasis on any of the words. 'I am OK.'

'Yes, I AM OK', Jennifer emphasised the 'AM', but immediately felt that this wasn't right. 'No, that sounds like I am telling myself that I am OK, but it is more than that, I don't need to tell myself, I know, I am OK, however wretched I might feel, however much hurt may emerge, it doesn't matter, I am OK, and I can take strength from that even though I cannot explain it at all.'

'I really hear you emphasising the OKness within yourself, Jennifer.' Laura did not feel any urge to want to qualify this, she wanted to accept and embrace Jennifer's experiencing warmly and with unconditional acceptance.

The counsellor could, in this moment, be carrying a sense of – yes, all very well, but there's still a lot of hurt to work through and this OKness is probably only temporary so I need to keep it in perspective. The person-centred counsellor will wholeheartedly accept the client's experience and will not seek to undermine it by trying to offer an angle that is coming from their own frame of reference. It is therapeutically helpful for clients to be allowed to experience what is present for them and for that experience to be honoured and valued unconditionally. When a client gives insight into their experience and the counsellor feels a response of 'yes but', then they are most likely outside of the client's frame of reference and need to go and deal with their own stuff.

Time had passed and the session was drawing to a close. 'I want to end on that, Laura, I feel strong and want to carry that with me. I know it won't last, most probably, but that's how I want to be for the moment.'

Laura respected this and they agreed to the usual time the following week. After Jennifer had gone Laura took time to just sit and reflect and to be with her own feelings. It had been another very intense session, and she had been struck by how forcefully she had experienced that urge to reach out and hold Jennifer, and how valuable that had been. And that sense of OKness had been palpable somehow, a real connection had developed between them in that session. She eventually noted this down whilst making a note in her own mind as to how much she had to reflect on in her next supervision session.

Supervision

'Jennifer has re-experienced being sexually abused by her father, of being penetrated, in fact she owned the fact that it was rape, and that seemed to have been quite a significant acknowledgement for her to make. Helped her recognise that she was helpless, not to be blamed, that it was forced on her. She also spoke about him talking to her, telling her how much she liked it, and everything. Horrible.'

'Horrible? Hard to listen to?'

'Somehow no, I think because I feel so strongly connected to Jennifer that whilst it is horrible I do feel I am in there. I don't have a sense of backing off at all.'

'OK. So it's horrible but you feel a strong sense of connection and of not backing off. You're there for her?'

'Yes, and particularly so in the last session where something really seemed to shift. I had a tremendous sense of a need to reach out to and hold Jennifer during one particular period of distress. And it seemed to be so timely, and somehow we came out of it more connected.'

'More connected. So I am wondering what was present for you when you reached out?'

'I can remember a sense of wanting to protect, and it was so strong. And it seemed to have coincided with Jennifer experiencing a tremendous need to be held, to be cared for, to be loved.'

'So you connected with her through an embrace in a moment when she was really wanting this. Had she voiced that need then?'

'No. It was a sense, an urge, that I had and I acted on.'

'And it seemed very helpful to Jennifer?'

'It did. She seemed to have really needed that response to her need to be cared for. Yet I had no logical reason for acting as I did, it just emerged in the moment.'

'Did you feel connected to Jennifer then in that moment?'

'Yes. It wasn't me in myself thinking "I need to do something". I know how false that can be, in fact I think of it as a kind of "false-congruence". No, this was a spontaneous urge that seemed to emerge out of my feeling very connected to Jennifer, even though she had not been saying much at all. I just somehow felt connected and was being very attentive to her.'

'An urge to protect. And how did Jennifer react?' Malcolm could sense a desire to explore this further. It somehow felt that there was more but he couldn't identify what it was. But something, somewhere, was nagging at him to pursue this a little more. He wanted to be sure that Laura's interpretation of her experience really matched what was present. He recognised the importance of helping supervisees to explore themselves when there may be incongruence present.

Merry (1999, p. 174) suggests that the emphasis in client-centred supervision should be on therapist congruence in the context of Rogers' 'necessary and sufficient conditions'. He goes on to draw the distinction that 'this stands in contrast to supervision practice in many other approaches to therapy (and sometimes in client-centred therapy) where client material forms the basis of supervision sessions, and discussion is limited to technical questions concerning the communication of empathic understanding, or the development of treatment plans and goals for therapy'.

'She said it was what she needed, that it was, how did she put it? That it was, yes, that it was what she needed and that she had felt very small and that the feelings had felt very big. She described them as a tidal wave.'

'She was very small, you mean in relation to the feelings, or she was connected with herself when she was very small?'

'She implied the former but I guess both.' Laura stopped and thought for a moment. 'There was something motherly about my reaction.'

'Motherly?'

'Yes, in my wanting to protect her, like I might have wanted to protect her if she was my own daughter.' As she said this Laura felt emotions rising in herself. 'Oh, something stirred in me saying that. I need to stay with this.'

'Mmmm, something about being motherly and protecting her as if she was your own daughter.'

Laura nodded. 'She's drawing the mother out of me, or am I over-identifying with her? Or am I simply experiencing feelings that anyone might feel for someone who needs to be cared for?' She sat for a moment and closed her eyes and tried to feel her way into her own experiencing. What did she feel towards

Jennifer? As she posed the question she could see Jennifer splitting into two, her as a child and her as an adult. 'I can see Jennifer as a child and as an adult and I am wondering if I feel differently towards them. I can see myself wanting maybe to mother the child and yet at that moment in the session the child side of Jennifer was not being talked about. I wasn't thinking of the child, but of Jennifer the woman sitting there in front of me. I wanted to mother Jennifer the adult. It was real but it wasn't a straight woman-to-woman or person-to-person response, was it? It had overtones of something else. Shit. It was such an intense time, and now I am left wondering what effect it had on Jennifer in the sense of how she experienced it given what was going on for me. And I don't know, other than that she said it had been timely and it left her feeling good. And it left me with a sense of OKness about everything, which I remember voicing. And Jennifer said how she felt stronger and we ended the session on her owning that and wanting to carry that out with her, whilst she was also recognising that it probably wouldn't last. So she wasn't losing perspective. But it was very intense, very powerful. But I am troubled by how much I may have been wanting to mother her, and I am also wondering why I need to be troubled because, so what, it was an intense time and I really want to own my reaction.'

'That sounds very affirming, you want to own your reaction. You felt a strong mothering urge to protect, you acted on it, it seemed to have been therapeutically valuable and it has left you feeling somehow closer to Jennifer and she is feeling stronger.'

'Yes, that sums it up. And hearing you say it like that leaves me feeling more assured about it all. But then, am I letting you rescue me here from any unease I have? I want to evaluate this from the standpoint of my own experiencing. Jennifer had gone silent and I don't know what that was all about, but it is likely to have been about her childhood. So she was probably engaging with thoughts, feelings, memories concerning her early life experience and probably linked to the sexual abuse. Oh, and her mother, her mother knew, she remembers seeing her in the doorway when she was out of body.' Laura spoke so factually as she added this last bit that Malcolm could have simply accepted it, but he didn't because it jumped out at him and he felt a reaction.

'What did the mother do?'

'Watch and walk away. She didn't do anything to stop it, at least that is Jennifer's memory. She has only had a few flashbacks I think of seeing her mother watching from the doorway.'

'Let me summarise what I am hearing, Laura, and see how you respond. Jennifer is silent, probably reconnecting with experiences linked to her being sexually abused by her father, and which also involves her mother watching and doing nothing. And you experience a strong motherly urge to protect her.'

'Yeah. Not surprising is it, when you say it like that.' Laura reflected for a moment. 'And I've remembered something else. Earlier in that last session Jennifer spoke of feeling betrayed and had quite a strong reaction to it, but that got lost somewhere. Somehow that theme didn't get explored further. What happened?' Laura thought for a moment. 'Yes, she spoke of feeling fragile, and then of being, how did she put it? On the edge of herself. Yes, and before that, when she spoke of feeling betrayed she had said something about her mother should have been there to protect her. And then I lived that out and yet it seemed to have been at a moment that was therapeutically helpful in some way, but I don't know what Jennifer was experiencing in that moment, and I really wish I did now. But that moment has gone.'

'So, it seems that your reaction was linked into the unexplored and unresolved issue of betrayal and not being protected, perhaps.'

Laura felt herself go quiet and she knew what was going on for her. It was suddenly very clear. 'It wasn't me trying to be her mother, it was me as a woman not wanting to own that her mother, a woman, could do nothing. It's a gender issue. Her father was a sexual abuser. He's a man and I don't have to defend him. But her mother is/was a woman, and I do have to defend womanhood. I say I have to, I mean that in this context I had to. I had to compensate for her mother. I wasn't trying to be her mother, I don't think, but I was trying to restore her faith in womanhood.'

'Her faith?' Malcolm knew the answer to his question before he asked it, but he needed to encourage Laura to own what was present for her.

'OK. Yeah. You're right. My faith. Shit. I could listen to her talking of her father abusing her, penetrating her, hurting her, leaving her feeling torn apart, and I could hold that. But her mother, watching from the doorway and doing nothing. Oh no. I didn't want to accept that. I didn't want to own that women, a woman, could do that. Shit! I need to clear this out, Malcolm. I can't let myself react like this to her mother as this is not going to go away. She hasn't talked about it yet, but she is bound to confront her mother. I have to be able to listen to it, and I can't let my reactions get in the way. Yet it does feel really helpful to have identified it and I wonder if this raised awareness is enough.'

The history of their supervision relationship has encouraged Laura to feel safe to explore her feelings openly with Malcolm. This is an important feature of effective supervision. Merry suggests that supervision 'provides opportunities for supervisees (counsellors) to experience a relationship that is free of threat, and is supportive and understanding so that they can explore non-defensively what the counselling process means to them, and how they experience themselves in relation to clients' (Merry, 1999, p. 140).

'What do you think?' Malcolm wanted to encourage Laura to trust her own prompting on this, she knew what she was experiencing and how difficult it felt.

'Part of me thinks, "therapy issue", and I will take it to therapy. And yet I also feel that now that I have, as it were, brought it to light, I think I will feel different and can be less inclined to react, I was going to say, as a woman. And yet that's ridiculous. I am a woman, I want to be a woman, and I want to support my client, who is also a woman, in resolving the trauma of being sexually abused by a man and betrayed/abandoned by a woman.'

'Sounds strong and clear.'

'Yeah. But I will take it to therapy. And I will carry into the sessions an awareness of the sensitivity that I have.' Laura stopped again for a moment. 'You know, I wonder if the reason we felt close after my holding Jennifer was somehow linked to her experiencing – and me experiencing – a sense of feminine solidarity. I wonder if, out of all of this, a real woman-to-woman, adult-to-adult moment emerged and, if so, I feel sure that it was therapeutically helpful.'

'Mmmm.' Malcolm nodded, happy to accept what Laura had said, but he was troubled still by something, and he was doing a reality check on himself because of being a man. 'I'm stuck with something Laura, and I don't think it is because I am a man, but I am open to that possibility so please say what you experience. We have focused on your reaction to Jennifer's mother and made sense of that. But what about her father? I am stuck with your implying something about being able to listen to Jennifer talk about what he did, and the contrast of that with your reaction to her mother. Am I now expressing man-to-man solidarity here, or is there something around, I don't know, the idea I have heard sometimes that essentially all men are abusers?'

Malcolm is using his own experience as a basis for exploring the issue being considered in supervision. He senses something but does not know quite what it is, but is happy to explore this with his supervisee in the context of their relationship in case it has relevance. This degree of openness and transparency by the supervisor provides for a broadly collaborative approach to supervision, recognising that it is not only the relationship between supervisee and client that is significant, but also the relationship between the supervisor and the material concerning their client that is being described in supervision by the supervisee.

'I don't see all men as abusers. I like men, though not all men obviously. Are you saying I could listen too easily to the parts about her father?'

'I'm not sure, but something like that, as if there is a kind of acceptance of his behaviour because he is a man, and that's what some men do.' Malcolm stopped. 'No. This could be my stuff here. I feel like I'm defending. But that doesn't mean there isn't something for you in all this as well. This will be a supervision issue for me, but I think it would be helpful to try to get clarity here as well.'

'I don't get a reaction of "your issue", I actually feel drawn to want to explore this as well. I do feel quite shocked by what I have been hearing. A few sessions back I remember Jennifer talking about how it hurt her, how she felt torn apart, and I did feel shock, a kind of jarring of my senses. I don't think I feel a sense of, well, "that's what men do". I feel shocked by what he did, her father – a single man, not every man. No, not every man.' Laura stopped again as an idea had come to mind, and it had taken her back to the issue with Jennifer's mother. 'I do think that maybe not addressing the experience of betrayal by her mother may have left me feeling, at some level, that I had betrayed her. Hence my need to protect may have been muddled in with a need to compensate. But with her father, no, I know that was just him. It was terrible, awful, it shouldn't have happened. And he betrayed her trust as well. Yet there is a difference, I think, between a man-to-woman and a woman-to-woman betrayal, and I guess man-to-man as well. It is something about there being some kind of fundamental gender solidarity, perhaps, I don't know. It is fascinating to explore.'

'Yes, I'm sure you are right. And it probably gets complicated when we add in sexual preference as this then adds another layer of solidarity. But maybe this is taking us away a bit from where we are at with Jennifer and her father.'

'How do you feel, as a man, listening to me talking about Jennifer's father?'

Malcolm hadn't expected that question, but felt good about it being asked by Laura. It said something about the mutuality of their relationship. 'A real mixture of sadness and anger, a compassion for them both, though I do feel more for Jennifer whilst I have a sense of the awful dilemma that her father is now in, or may be in if he is uncomfortable about the sexual abuse of his daughter. I am aware that as a man I am affected when I hear about what men do, and particularly when it is used to somehow make collectively sweeping statements about all men. So I am aware that I own my reactions and I need to let go of them in order to attend fully to what you are bringing to me. When my reactions get in the way of me listening to you, then I have a problem. I am not experiencing this difficulty. I want to be there wholeheartedly for you as you seek to help and support Jennifer through her awful memories and the effect it is having, and will have, on her family. I hate what he has done, but I do not really have such sense of him other than what you are telling me. So I have a partial view of him which I know is incomplete, and I know that my real focus is for you, Jennifer and the relationship you are creating, and how I then experience that when you bring it to me. I hadn't meant to say quite that much.'

'I'm glad you have, it kind of makes more of you visible to me and I appreciate that. I am struck with the thought that all this seemed to bring Jennifer and me closer, and it feels like it has done the same for us. An intriguing bit of parallel processing.' With that Laura glanced at her watch. 'Time has passed and I need to talk about another of my clients. I don't feel I have touched on everything I could have done, but I think the other things can hold.'

'Was there anything else?'

'I had wanted to talk about Jennifer feeling dirty and developing what seems a not unreasonable washing obsession, but she didn't talk about that last time and maybe that is something we can come back to another time. It doesn't feel pressing, I guess I just want to flag it up. I don't like going away knowing that I haven't at least mentioned what I wanted to say.'

They drew the emphasis on Jennifer to a close and moved on to another of Laura's clients.

Points for discussion

- Was Laura right to say that Jennifer did not have to get clean?
- What specifically makes the person-centred approach an effective method for helping people resolve the memories of traumatic experiences?
- How do you react to the idea that a client has had an out-of-body experience? Can you accept their experience, and if not, what stops you?
- What feelings and reactions became present for you as you read Jennifer retelling her childhood experiences of sexual abuse and rape? How can you ensure they would not obstruct the quality of your empathy for a client telling you of similar experiences?
- In the last session the theme of betrayal did not get addressed as fully as it might have done. Why was this? Would you have handled it differently?
- What do you think happened to explain the timeliness of Laura reaching out to Jennifer and holding her in that last session?
- What are your views on the gender discussion that developed during supervision?
- How do you feel affected by Jennifer's disclosure of obsessive behaviour and what might you have sought to explore about this in supervision?

CHAPTER 8

Counselling session 46

'Really feels like autumn now, leaves are changing and there's a real damp cold in the air tonight. Glad it's nice and warm in here.' Jennifer was taking her coat off and settling into the chair in Laura's counselling room.

'Yes, it feels like the end of October now, doesn't it?'

'And a time for reflection, moving into the winter months. Wasn't the end of October the old Celtic New Year, a time of transition from the old to the new? Seems to me that is where I am at the moment. So much to come to terms with, so many feelings and thoughts, and so busy. I am aware as well that I am pushing stuff away and I know that isn't good, but it is getting me through at the moment.'

Laura nodded, 'Busy time, lots going on, thoughts of transition from the old to the new, so I am wondering how you want to use the session this evening?'

Laura decides not to engage in a discussion over the Celtic New Year, but rather highlights briefly what has been said and opens the session up for Jennifer to choose her focus. An example of non-directivity, such a crucial feature of person-centred working.

'It feels that my time here is really precious, and there is so much I need to come to terms with and, I don't know, work out what the hell to do with. I still experience waves of feelings when I think of the past, of my father and what he did to me, and of my mother, and I really need to make sense of it. I need to talk to them, and I realise I have to now talk to them both. I need to have an answer to the "why?" and the "why me?" that is in my head. But I am also aware of there being a lot going on for me at work at the moment, and I have to make some choices around my work and I really would value using time this evening to talk about that.' Jennifer genuinely felt caught between wanting to continue exploring her past, but she knew that work issues were very much to the fore.

Laura responded by acknowledging the dilemma, and suggested that really it was for Jennifer to decide what she felt to be most pressing, that the session was Jennifer's and that she was happy to listen, respond and help her explore whatever she wanted to bring. Jennifer thought about it but realised that she really did need to talk about her work. She described the changes in the organisation and the possible change of role for her. Much of the rest of the session continued on this theme, with Jennifer seeking a clearer sense of her own thoughts and feelings regarding her options and the likely effects of what she might decide to do.

The conversation moved on towards the end of the session. Jennifer had realised that whilst she did want to take on more responsibility at work, she actually felt that the time was not right. It was leaving her feeling angry that her past was making it difficult for her to take what she felt would be a positive step for her in the present.

'If it hadn't happened, if I didn't feel that the next – oh I don't know how long – the next few months are going to be dominated by my resolving being sexually abused, I'd go for it. Damn it, why should he fuck up my life now. Fucked. That's what I feel, fucked.' As she said this Jennifer could feel a tremendous surge of anger rising up inside herself. 'Fucked then, fucked now.' She spat the words out. I just want to get on with my life. But I can't, can I? I've got to get my head sorted out first, and whilst I feel I've started, I'm sure I have a long way to go. Bastard.'

'I feel the anger, fucked then, fucked now, just wanting to get on with your life.' Laura spoke with force in her voice, seeking to reflect the tone of Jennifer's voice.

'I do, and I don't want what he did to me messing it all up. I feel messed up, sometimes I really feel as though I'm going crazy. I don't feel normal sometimes. I sit there in the bath and catch myself washing myself between my legs, realising I have been doing it for some time but with no sense of time passing. I lose myself in washing, trying to get clean, and it's his fault. It's his fucking fault.' Jennifer's voice got stronger and again the anger was palpable. Her fists were clenched and her jaw was clamped tight. 'I'm going to get over this, Laura, I'll be damned if I'm going to let him destroy my life.'

Laura responded to where Jennifer had left off. 'Determined, you're going to come through this. You're not going to let him destroy your life.'

'Bloody well not. Shit, it actually feels good to be angry. Feels like I have a lot of energy.' Jennifer could feel a lot of strength in her body although she could feel the tension in her muscles as well. 'I'm going to need it.'

'Mmmm, going to need all that angry energy.'

'You know, the more I think about it now, the more I question whether I should duck out of this opportunity at work. Dammit, I've earned it. I know we just spent the whole session talking about it, but somehow, feeling like I do now, I really feel I want to go for it, and stuff him. It's like getting angry has helped me connect with the part of me that wants to succeed, wants to prove something.'

'Prove something?' Laura wondered what and to whom, but she held back from saying this, preferring to leave it open for Jennifer.

'Prove that I AM good enough, that I, that I . . . .' Jennifer could feel emotions rising and tears in her eyes. 'Shit.' She shook her head.

Laura waited for Jennifer to speak, sensing correctly that a process was running for her and that she needed to be uninterrupted to allow herself to go with it.

Empathic sensitivity should allow the counsellor to recognise a working silence, and when it occurs the person-centred counsellor will trust the client to be focusing on what is most important. The process is trusted and the counsellor maintains a state of attentiveness and an attitude of warm acceptance.

'Something about feeling unclean, not good enough and having to prove myself, but thinking that I can't. That's from the past. I've got to break free of it, Laura, I'm going for this new role and I'm going to do it for me.'

'You really want to break free from feeling unclean and not good enough . . . .' Once again Laura did not have a chance to finish her empathic response as Jennifer continued.

'I am me. I am not dominated by what he did. I am not dirty. I am not messed up. I am going to get on with my life and do what I want, and not because of what happened in the past.' She paused. 'That feels good. OK. I am going to talk to my boss tomorrow and start things moving. And I will deal with my past, but if I am doing what I want to do now I think I will be stronger.'

Jennifer really felt the strength in what she was saying, and it felt good to affirm to herself, and to Laura, what she felt, what she thought. Yes, she thought, I need this, I need focus, I need direction. I know I have to look back and sort stuff out, but I want to look forwards as well. Though she knew deep within her there was uncertainty and that sense of feeling disturbed by what she was remembering from her past, she also felt a need to get things in perspective. She felt, at least in this moment, that she could do that.

'Sounds like you have made up your mind.' Laura was aware that it could be too soon, but then it might not be. Who was she to know what was best for Jennifer? She trusted that Jennifer would do what she needed to do, and she wasn't going to start questioning that, placing doubt where this was not what Jennifer wished to communicate to her. She wanted to convey an encouraging warm acceptance. She smiled. 'You're going to go for it, and we can use the time here to focus on whatever you need to work on, yes?'

'Yes. OK. So, same time next week, but the week after I am away a couple of evenings mid-week and then taking some annual leave. So I won't be able to see you then.'

'Fine. So, I'll see you next week.'

She really shifted once she got in touch with her anger, Laura thought as she pondered the session afterwards. All the careful weighing up of what she should do at work, all the logic, and then getting in touch with that anger released a determination to go for it. She hoped it would work out. She knew that it might not, but she also knew how important it was to allow her client to make her own choices. In truth, she, Laura, didn't know what was best for Jennifer. She was pleased that she hadn't been tempted to caution her, or to suggest she needed to think about it more, and run the risk of sliding into some protective mother figure as she had explored in the last supervision session.

Counselling session 47

Jennifer started the session describing the changes at work and how she felt about them. She was to take more responsibility in her role and take on extra management duties. This felt good and whilst it was already clear that it would mean more work, she felt she could cope with it. She was aware of being a little apprehensive, but also excited by it all.

'I want to ....' There was a sudden loud bang outside. Jennifer felt herself jump. 'What was that?'

'Fireworks, it's 5th November!'

'Yes, but it sounded very close.' Jennifer took a moment to regain her thoughts. 'I want to say some more about feeling disturbed by the memories of the past. It's strange, I can really push it aside and get on with things, and then something happens and I am aware of feeling weak, but that's not the right word, or at least it's only part of it. It's that feeling fragile again, feeling like I'm a bit blurry, kind of fuzzy. It's like it creeps over me and leaves me feeling cold and trembly. And I seem powerless to stop it when it happens. My heart seems to race and I feel like I need fresh air. I don't know, I can just feel really weird.'

'That sounds very descriptive, Jennifer, fuzzy, blurred, disturbed, cold, trembling.'

Jennifer nodded, 'And I want to add the word "uneasy" to the list. And sometimes, well often, when it happens at home, I find myself thinking of having a drink, and sometimes I do, and it helps, but I know it isn't the answer, but it does help. Makes me feel warm and it seems to lift that unease. It's a horrible feeling, but I really don't want to keep using alcohol to cope with it. I know where that could take me. And it isn't all the time, but sometimes, usually if I am alone. When Ian's there I can tell him what is happening for me and we just talk and he holds me, and it passes. But when he's not there it is really hard to shake it off. It scares me, Laura, I don't want these feelings, but they are there.'

'Scary to have those feelings and to react to them by having a drink, yeah?'

'Yeah. Thinking about it gives me the creeps.'

'You experience it now, talking about it?'

'Not as bad, but sort of. It's the uneasiness I am feeling right now. Just feeling disturbed, like something isn't right. And I know what has happened to cause this, but knowing that doesn't take it away. It's there, inside me, and I want it to go away.' She looked up at Laura. 'I wish you could take it away.'

'Like you, I wish I could take it away.' Laura felt the urge to say more but stopped herself, feeling that what she had said conveyed her caring and wanting to help Jennifer. She felt it would perhaps help her to stay with her experience and perhaps that would help her to release some of the feelings, or connect with them to explore a little further. She didn't know what would happen next. But she sat, maintaining eye contact with Jennifer, and quietly said, 'It would be so good not to have that unease deep inside yourself.'

In making this comment, flowing out of the empathic contact that Laura is experiencing, a profound sense of deep connection is established within Jennifer. She finds herself moving towards a connection with her feeling of unease and, as a result, enters into a dissociated state that is associated with this experience – feeling out-of-body. Such moments of deep connection, however disturbing the experience, tend to foster growth and movement. Rogers wrote of 'moments of movement' which he described in terms of being moments in therapy when actual growth seems to occur.

Silence. As she sat there Jennifer could feel the unease growing and expanding from inside the pit of her stomach. It expanded across her body, up her chest, down into her hips and thighs, up to her shoulders and into her arms, further down into her legs. It reached into her head and she felt very strange, kind of floating and buzzy. She felt like she was not really in her body, as though she had stepped out of it. She realised that she had, that she was actually looking down on the session, or at least, looking over her own head towards Laura. Yet she was still sitting there and she was aware she had her eyes closed, but somehow had them open at the same time. She knew this sensation, it was what had happened when she was being sexually abused by her father, and had happened that time when she had been making love with Ian. Somehow, though, she felt less unease now, as though she had stepped away from it, left it behind. Yes, she kind of knew she had left it behind, left it in her body somehow. And yet it wasn't. It was like it was still with her but now it felt different, like it was somehow OK to be there. It was like she didn't feel she had to fight it anymore.

Laura was quite unaware of what had happened to Jennifer. She had noticed Jennifer close her eyes as she had spoken those last words, and had noticed a slight shudder as she sat there, but now she seemed to be just sitting back in the chair. Her head rolled forward and Laura thought she had drifted off to sleep or had fainted, and just as she began to react, Jennifer jolted, opened her eyes and blinked, looking around, looking like she was trying to focus.

'What happened?' Laura asked.

'I-I'm not sure, at least, I know what it felt like.' She reached for the water. It felt cool and somehow reassuring as she felt it flow down her throat and into her stomach. Helped her to somehow feel she was back in herself.

'Take your time, it looked like it was a bit of a shock.' Laura waited for Jennifer to continue.

'I really connected with that sense of unease, I mean, I really felt I had connected with it, just held in it and it was strange, but I felt sort of out of myself again, like the unease was there and I was standing next to it, but it was within me as well. It's hard to describe, but it felt like something shifted inside of me, as if I saw something of myself, experienced myself in some new way. Oh God, is this making any sense?'

'Can I say how I am hearing you?'

'Yes, that would be helpful.'

'OK. You connected with the unease but somehow felt yourself to be both beside it and it was part of you. And as a result you have felt some kind of shift, though I am unclear what that last bit means to you.'

'I'm feeling somehow a bit more connected up. I don't know how to describe it.' Jennifer stopped and thought about it for a moment. 'Yes,' she finally said, 'yes, it's like, if you can imagine a jigsaw and you have a piece and you don't know where it goes. Well, somehow the unease seems to feel like a piece that has found its place, like it has become familiar and somehow OK. I don't think I have to fight it anymore, but I'm really not sure what I mean by that.'

'You don't feel you have to fight the unease any more? You know where it fits in? Kind of accepted it?'

'Kind of feels more than acceptance but I don't have a word for it. Like it's OK. It's OK. I don't have to push it away. I think I've been doing that for years, but somehow it's OK. Something's happened to me, Laura, I feel different, and it was in that moment of experience, but I know I still can't really make sense of it.' Jennifer knew something had changed profoundly but it was so hard to put into words. But she sensed that Laura had appreciated what she was trying to say, and that felt good, and it felt reassuring as well.

'You feel different and it is somehow more than acceptance.'

Laura holds her empathic focus, keeping her response simple and to the point, allowing Jennifer to continue to explore what she is experiencing.

Jennifer thought about it again. Different, more than acceptance. The words went through her mind as she sat. An image came to her mind and she could see herself in a sense embracing her unease, embracing it, taking it into herself, but freely, openly, with warm acceptance. Yes. 'It's like I've embraced the unease, accepted it as part of me and somehow as a result it has lost its power over me. I feel like I know more of who I am. It's like I am building this picture of myself and my experiences, particularly from the past, but now I am aware of them consciously and something is changing as a result.'

Laura nodded. 'So becoming more consciously aware of your past and of yourself now is causing this change, and it involves embracing your unease.'

'And that unease goes back to the sexual abuse, Laura, that undermined me and that's what I have to overcome, and it feels like I am moving in the right direction.'

'Mmmm. Overcoming the unease that resulted from being sexually abused and feeling undermined, and now you have a sense of moving in the right direction.'

'It wasn't just the abuse from my father that did it, you know, and I feel different as I say this, but it was my mother abandoning me. I felt worthless, undeserving of help. Somehow I can see that now and I feel sad about it, and angry about it, but I can also look at it and acknowledge it.'

Laura was listening closely to what Jennifer was saying and what struck her was the way that Jennifer was speaking. It felt like she was able to put things into a different perspective, as though she was in a sense disidentifying from the effects of some of her experiences. The effects were there, she could see them and experience them, but she wondered if she had freed up her identity from them in some way.

'You look lost in thought, Laura.'

'Mmm? Oh, sorry, yes, it was what you were saying and how you are being, it left me thinking about how it feels like you have freed up, or in some sense released, your identity to some degree from the effects of the past. Like you were disidentifying from parts of yourself. I'm not saying that's how it is, but it is where my thoughts went just now.'

What is happening for Jennifer is that she seems to no longer be focusing her identity so strongly in parts of herself that developed in response to, and as part of the coping mechanism for, the experience of sexual abuse in childhood. It is not that she is pushing them away, but in a sense has embraced them as parts of herself and in that act of embracing or accepting them, has integrated them in such a way that they are less of a dominant feature within her structure of self. They are still there, but her focus is elsewhere, as though the actualising tendency has found new areas of her structure of self to work through. So rather than her tendency to grow and seek greater satisfaction remaining centred in the damaged and traumatised parts of herself that relate back to her childhood experience, it now has focus in a more positive and congruent sense of self.

'Yes. But I can't really explain it. I feel I can sit here now and I know that I drifted a little while ago, but now I feel more compact, more centred in me, and it is a me that feels different.'

'More compact, more centred.' These two words had somehow stood out to Laura as she listened and she reflected them back.

Jennifer nodded and sat in silence, thinking about it, and then feeling unsure what to think about. Somehow it made sense, but she didn't know where to go with it next. It felt like she had reached a conclusion to something, although it didn't feel final, but more like completing a step or a stage. Had she come to terms with her past? Had she? She felt unsure about that. She knew she didn't have all the memories. And she knew that she was, or had been, still coping with that unease with alcohol. Yet now she felt different. Would it hold? As she sat there now she certainly didn't feel like she had any attraction for alcohol, but that was now, being with Laura and feeling as she did. What would happen when she was home alone. Yet, as she had these thoughts, she was surprised not to feel anxious about it. That was different. But she also felt wary of being overconfident. She suddenly had a sense of time, and of having been sitting there for some time.

'You looked absolutely lost in thought there.'

Jennifer smiled. 'I was. All sorts of things. Wondering how much I have come to terms with things, wondering whether alcohol would still have the same attraction if I feel that unease creeping up on me again. Lots of questions, but no real answers.'

'Mmmm. Often how it is, lots of questions, no real answers.'

'I guess I'm not sure what I want to talk about now. I feel like I have got somewhere and now I'm sitting here wondering what to say, wondering what I want to use the rest of the time for. I don't feel an urge to talk about anything in particular, I feel strangely at ease with myself.'

'At ease. Is that something you want to explore?'

Jennifer thought for a moment. 'Yes, it is sort of unusual, at least, I do feel at ease but this feels different somehow, more kind of, I don't know, calmer somehow.'

'So a feeling of calmness?'

'Yes. It feels like a stillness, like I could almost just sit quietly and be with it and it would be nourishing.'

'So, stillness to just sit quietly with, and a sense that nourishment would emerge out of it.'

'Yes. I'd actually like to do that.'

'Sure, what sit and be with the stillness?'

'Yes. And I think I want to just close my eyes.'

'Fine. How do you feel about me closing my eyes too and seeking to be in stillness as well, or would you prefer that I keep my eyes open and wait for you to come out when you feel ready.'

'I'd like us both to be still, maybe for, I don't know, maybe ten minutes. Just be in silence together.'

'OK. I'll leave it for you to let me know when you want to move on from it, but I'll keep an eye on the time in case you overrun, and perhaps say when ten minutes have passed?'

'Yes, that sounds good.'

Periods of shared silence or of meditation within a counselling session can be extremely helpful, and can add another dimension to the shared experience of the therapeutic relationship. Jennifer has not been directed to do this, it has emerged from her own sense of what her needs are. Laura has been attentive to this and her responses have really been to clarify what

> Jennifer wants. She takes responsibility for the time-keeping, taking this concern away from Jennifer, and therefore allowing her to be free of any 'time-watching' anxiety.

Jennifer closed her eyes and took a couple of deep breaths. It felt right to be doing this, like sharing in a kind of silent meditation. She wasn't sure what to think about, and then a word came into her mind, something that Laura had said – 'disidentifying'. Yes, disidentifying, felt like letting go of parts of herself that she no longer needed to be. It reminded her of a meditation technique she had come across years ago, of calmly affirming how you have a body, but in essence are not your body, that you have feelings and emotions, but in essence you are more than they are, that you have thoughts, but you are more than your thoughts. She thought about her body. Yes, it had been abused, and she hated the images and the feelings that were around from that time. But that was her body then, not now. The thought came to her mind that the body she had today has not been sexually abused. Her body as a mature woman had not gone through that experience, though it had been a horribly significant feature of its early development. She didn't need to wash her body now to try to make it clean, make it *feel* clean.

Feelings. Yes, she carried feelings from the past, strong feelings, and she had feelings now, about her father's denial, and feelings towards her mother, and wonderings as to how she would react when she is confronted with the past. Lots of feelings, but am I more than my feelings? Feelings shape me, and the way I feel about myself as a result of how I interpret experiences. She thought about the unease she had experienced, and how she was now affirming herself at work. Feelings are strong, they can fire me up and deflate me back down, but they are not *me*. I can think about my feelings as well as experience them. So am I my thoughts?

Jennifer continued her train of thought, deciding that yes, she had thoughts, she had a mind, she used her mind, but there was still the question of who the 'she' was that was using her mind. I have feelings, thoughts, bodily sensations, and they can be pleasurable and satisfying, and they can be painful and make me feel less of myself. But they are not me. So who am I?

The question hung in her thoughts and she had no answer, other than somehow there seemed to be a strength in this unanswered question. It was like she didn't need to know who she was, but it was more important to know who she wasn't. And yet she also wanted to know who the 'she' was that she experienced herself to be, that was more than her body, feelings and thoughts. Yet she didn't feel anxious at the thought, she remained quite calm and relaxed about it. Kind of meditative as she continued to sit, allowing herself to drift away from thoughts, feelings and sensations in her body, finding instead a deep and satisfying stillness.

Laura meanwhile was sitting reflecting on what stillness meant for her and seeking at the same time not to completely let go of being aware that she was there as Jennifer's counsellor. Yet it felt good to just have this personal stillness within the context of the therapeutic relationship. She wasn't sure what meaning it would have for Jennifer, in truth, she hadn't a clue, and that was OK. She didn't need to know. She accepted the reality of the moment and stayed open to her own experiencing. She reflected back over the sessions and the experiences that she and Jennifer had shared in recent months, particularly since she began to reconnect with the memories of being sexually abused.

She regarded counselling, therapy, psychotherapy – she felt the terms were interchangeable – as a journey and that over time changes took place without it always being clear that any particular occasion led to a specific change. She knew that holding the core conditions would have a therapeutic effect, and she felt sure that over time Jennifer was sorting and sifting through her regained memories and finding ways of making sense of it all, for herself, and in ways that were psychologically helpful for her. Clearly, she was becoming more self-affirming, and there did seem to be an increasing degree of self-acceptance emerging as well, which is such an important factor in therapeutic change.

Laura didn't want to tie herself up in endless speculation, rather she felt she wanted to hold a feeling of honouring and celebrating the journey so far, and the promise of further growth for Jennifer towards an increasingly satisfying and less negatively conditioned sense of self. And she wanted to celebrate her own part in helping Jennifer so far. It felt good to feel she was making a positive difference in someone else's life.

The time. Laura glanced at her watch. Twelve minutes, they'd overrun. She looked over to Jennifer who still had her eyes shut and seemed to be ever so slightly smiling as she sat there, looking quite serene and untroubled. It was lovely to see. 'Twelve minutes have passed, Jennifer, but come out of it in your own time and in your own way.' She noticed a slight nod from Jennifer so she sat back in the chair and waited.

Jennifer took a deep breath. She felt refreshed. 'Thanks for that. It felt good. I seemed to find that stillness and it helped me see things in a different perspective. It felt healing. It was a good way to draw the session to a close. I want to take that sense of stillness and healing with me.'

Jennifer affirmed what she had been pondering on during the silence, and asked Laura what she had experienced. She described her sense of wanting to honour and celebrate Jennifer's journey. Jennifer then acknowledged that she knew she was only part way along it and that she still had aspects of her past to come to terms with, and the whole subject of resolving her experiences with her parents, but she said she felt that at this moment she was on top of it and wanted to hold on to that.

The person-centred counsellor will want to leave the client free to decide whether or not to disclose what they have experienced during their quiet time, and will only disclose their own experience if requested to do so.

Jennifer confirmed again before she left that she would not be coming for two weeks.

Laura pondered on the session, and was once again amazed at the twists and turns that the therapeutic journey involved. She had not expected the session to develop as it had, but was glad that she worked in a way that allowed the client to direct things. It felt natural, organic, and she liked the not knowing. The next session? Who knows, she thought to herself. Who knows what will emerge? One thing she was sure about was that she should remain ready for anything. Jennifer might still be experiencing what had emerged for her this evening, but then maybe other experiences would disrupt that. She knew from experience of working with clients with similar experiences how fast things could change, how memories could surface and provoke a completely different set of experiences in a person to what was previously present. She acknowledged to herself that she wanted Jennifer to move through and on from her past, but she also realised that it could take time, that she was still being troubled by the memories, that she was drifting out-of-body at times and that it wasn't so long ago that she was experiencing dissociation in the sessions. But this had been quite an optimistic session in the sense that it had left Jennifer in a strong place within herself, a place that perhaps her actualising tendency was taking her towards as she came to terms with her past.

Counselling session 48

Jennifer began the session by describing how the feelings from the previous session had stayed with her for a few days, and how good it had been to know that that place within herself existed. However, she had had a bad weekend and whilst she had got through the following week, it had not been easy, her feelings and mood had fluctuated a lot. The problem she was experiencing was that the memories that were present for her were now bringing with them distinctive feelings, and she was finding these extremely difficult to deal with. She had also wet the bed on a couple of occasions, something she knew she did as a child, but hadn't done as an adult in years. That seemed to happen on nights when vivid memories re-emerged in her dreams, which felt like nightmares.

'I said before how I was aware of him, on me, in me, and when I was here that time saying how it hurt, well, that was what I experienced in that strange state I got into, but it also seemed distant afterwards, or at least, not so much distant as somehow not so real again. But now the memories come with really clear feelings and experiences. It's been so bad sometimes that it has made me physically sick.'

'Sounds as though it has all become much more real to you, much more complete somehow.' Laura sought to empathise with the sense of what was happening rather than reflect back what Jennifer had said specifically, reflecting her sense that the past was carrying much more of the experience within Jennifer's awareness in the present.

'It's like I'm experiencing it for real. I'm not looking on, I'm not remembering something as if it is somehow apart from me. Now it is present, real, here and now.'

'Sounds as though it has been a big change. Very much more in the here and now.'

Laura acknowledges the change but does not want to end her empathic response with this acknowledgement. She puts this first and finishes with a more direct empathic response to Jennifer's description of it being 'more in the here and now'. This style of response reduces the risk of directing the client away from her focus yet offers the opportunity for the counsellor to empathise with what she is sensing as the unvoiced process for the client.

'Big change. I guess it had to happen, but it's horrible. And it's much more graphic, I mean, *much* more graphic.' She shuddered.

'Looks like you are revolted by how graphic it has become, your body certainly is reacting.'

'All of me is reacting. I can remember what it was like waiting for him to come to my room. He didn't every night, I never knew, but I sense that I always expected him. I hated going to bed. I still feel that unease, and it has got worse now that I'm having these memories. I mean, they are now with me all the time, but some nights I really do seem to relive it, not just remember it, actually feel as though it is happening.'

Laura nodded, 'As though it is actually happening.' She was aware that her jaw had tightened. Her heart went out to Jennifer. God, what she is going through, and she felt her feelings towards Jennifer's father cut in. She acknowledged them but pushed them aside, as Jennifer continued.

'I'm lying there, the sheets pulled up. I'm on my side, I could never lie on my back to go to sleep, never. Never could and still can't, but only now I realise why. I'd hear the door open and he'd come in, quietly, talking softly, saying things like "Where's my special little girl?", "Daddy's come to show you how much he loves little Jenny". His voice, I can hear it so clearly, always calling me "his little Jenny". Now I also know why I always insist everyone calls me Jennifer, I hate it when it is shortened to Jenny. Ughh!' Jennifer shook her head and Laura could see her body tense as she said it. Her reaction was very present and visible.

'I can see the tension in you, and the revulsion, as you say that.'

'Feels horrible. I can feel the tension. I'd lie there, hardly daring to breathe. I'd close my eyes and huddle up in a ball. He'd begin by being very gentle with me. He'd come in under the covers and hold me, telling me what a beautiful little girl I was and how he was going to make me feel special. He kept using that word "special". Special, special, special. I hate it.' Jennifer began to sob. 'I hate it.'

'You hate it now.' Laura was aware that by adding the word now she was also encouraging a contrast to how Jennifer might have felt then.

'Hate it now.' Jennifer could feel herself reliving those experiences. Part of her had liked to be told she was special, but she had also been so scared. She didn't feel she understood. Being special, but it hurt and she had to do horrible things to be special.

'Hate it now.' Laura just reflected back softly, aware that Jennifer seemed to be focused very much in some kind of remembering and re-experiencing. She did not want to disturb her process.

'I was confused, I didn't understand. It was good to be special. It was nice to be held, to be hugged. At first it felt warm, it felt safe, and sometimes that was all that happened. Sometimes it wasn't any more than that. I can remember that. But not every time. And I don't understand that. Was he fighting himself? Did he change his mind sometimes? I don't know. I don't know.' Jennifer was shaking her head again.

'So sometimes he only held you and that felt good, but other times other things happened.'

Laura keeps it open, not being specific, not wanting to direct Jennifer to anything specific. She senses that Jennifer is going to describe what happened more clearly and she really wants her to choose her own way of saying it, her own emphasis, and in her own order.

'I liked being held, Laura. Was that so bad?'

Laura felt it important to affirm to Jennifer that it was not bad to want to be held. 'No, it can be good to feel held. We all like to feel held. But it wasn't always just being held.'

A direct question and Laura appropriately empathises with Jennifer's need for a direct answer. She gives it, and she also adds to this in order to keep the context visible.

'No.' A pause. 'Yes, I like to feel held, but it was/is so confusing. Even now with Ian I like to be held but it is hard to really let myself go, to really lose myself in being held, because something in me seems to keep me tense and holding back.'

'Something keeps you tense and holds you back.'

'Yeah, like I can't risk giving myself to being held, not really, completely. I always thought I did but now I've come to realise that I don't. And I think that's linked to drinking. It takes that tension out. It helps me let go, but it isn't real. It isn't me really letting go. It's the alcohol. And I don't want that. I want to be held and know that it is, that it is . . . .' Jennifer began sobbing again.

Laura sensed that it was in response to what she had been trying to say, so she reflected back questioningly, and softly, 'That it is?'

Jennifer spoke very quietly, Laura really had to listen hard to hear what she said. 'Safe.'

'You want to be held and know that it is safe.' Dammit, Laura thought, the moment she said it, I've put the phrase together for her, and it should have been for her to have said it.

Jennifer was nodding. Yes, she wanted to be able to feel safe. She wanted to get rid of the memory, the expectation, the fear, the . . . , the, the everything. 'Just to be held and to feel completely safe, and that I could just lose myself in that feeling of being held close and loved. Oh God, I want that feeling, Laura, I so want that feeling. And I've felt it here, I felt it when you held me here. I didn't experience any of this holding back in myself. But with Ian – I guess because he's a man – I find it so hard. And I don't want to be like that, I really don't. And I don't want to drink myself into it.'

'You really want that experience of being held close and loved, but it is so hard, even with Ian.'

Jennifer was nodding.

'You really don't want to feel you have to hold yourself back, and you don't want to use alcohol.'

Jennifer shook her head. She had closed her eyes.

'And there are things I won't do with Ian, and that's because of the past. I mean, oral sex. I can't. I just can't.' She went silent and pale. Laura respected the silence, but said quietly, 'That's something you just can't do.'

'He made me do it sometimes.'

Laura guessed that Jennifer was back to talking about her father.

'Made you do it.'

Jennifer nodded. 'Makes me feel sick thinking about it. Said it was what little girls did, and that how it was a really grown-up thing to do. He used to make all these horrible noises, and he'd come in my mouth. And it was awful, just awful.' The tears streamed down Jennifer's cheeks. She could feel herself gagging at the memory of it, the taste was in her mouth again, sticky, salty, hot, horrible. She could never get the taste away. She drank some water, it helped a little but it was difficult to swallow. 'I think I hated that the most. It was horrible, just horrible.' As Jennifer was speaking Laura had reached out her hand and taken Jennifer's hand in hers. As she continued to speak her grip tightened on Laura's hand.

'It was so horrible, Laura, and I know it can be really wonderful with someone you love. But I can't, I just can't. And I've explained why now to Ian. He seems to understand, but I don't want my past spoiling what we have, or could have.' Jennifer collapsed into floods of tears. She tried to speak but the words didn't come out. She loved Ian so much and she desperately didn't want to ruin it. As the tears eased she managed to get the words out, but slowly, and stutteringly.

'He-made-me-swallow-it. Told me that was what you had to do.' She closed her eyes as she felt the tears well up and a burning feeling rise up in her throat.

'Oh God, I think I'm going to be sick.' Jennifer got up and went out to the toilet. Jennifer heard Laura call out, asking if she was OK, if she could do anything, if she needed her. 'No, it's OK,' she replied. She wasn't actually sick, the reflex hadn't gone down into her stomach, but she could feel the burning in her throat. She felt quite weak as she came back a few minutes later. Laura had topped up her glass of water. Jennifer gratefully drank from it again, this time it went down a little easier, feeling cool against her throat.

'How are you feeling?'

'Weak and wobbly. Oh. I can relive that experience so easily at the moment, Laura, like it is so close. So very close.'

Jennifer lapsed into silence, She felt drained, utterly drained. 'Sorry, but I feel wiped out just at the moment. I need to just sit quietly I think.' She continued to sip the water. After a short while she continued. 'How do I cope with this? I mean, I can't get rid of what happened, but how do I live with it?'

'I don't know how you will find a way to live with it, Jennifer, but people find their own ways, and you'll find your way. In a way it is good that you are staying aware when you remember it now, and not going out-of-body or dissociating in the session. But I really hear that question that must be eating away at you, "how do I live with it?".'

'I don't think I went out-of-body with the oral sex, Laura, I think that was only when he was inside me, that is when he was inside my vagina, when he raped me. But I can remember that experience now as well, and much more clearly and vividly.'

Laura nodded.

'I have to find a way to live with it. I feel so used, so dirty sometimes. I mean, I know that who I am today isn't who I was then, but I know as well that it was me and that it has affected me, shaped me, left me with all kinds of feelings about myself. And I know I'm learning, discovering new ways of being, but it feels like a battle sometimes. It really does. And sitting here now I just feel like all the strength has been drained out of me, like someone's pulled out the plug and it's just swirled away.'

'Drained, yet knowing you have to find a way to live with it and discover new ways of being. It's one hell of a battle.'

Jennifer took a deep breath. 'Yeah. It is. And I'm going to survive this and come through it. It feels horrible just now, and I know I'm in a completely different place to where I was two weeks ago, but what happened then was real too, and I take strength from that. You know what it feels like?'

Laura didn't and replied, 'No, what does it feel like?'

'Like I've been dropped in shit, in that runny kind of shit you get on farms, covered in it and yet I know as well that there is more to me than the shit. That it will wash away. That I can remove the stench. But I don't think I'll ever feel really clean. And that feels ....' Jennifer swallowed. 'That feels very sad.' Her eyes watered as she said it but she held her eye contact with Laura.

Laura felt a huge wave of emotion sweep through her as she looked back into Jennifer's very watery eyes. She could feel the sadness rising up in her too and her own eyes watering. She allowed her own tears to trickle down her cheeks.

Seeing Laura's tears somehow gave Jennifer strength. She didn't understand it, couldn't make sense of it, didn't actually try. But it felt somehow confirming to see Laura's reaction. Made her sadness more acceptable. Yes, more acceptable. It was OK to feel sad. She had a right to feel sad. It made others feel sad. But she didn't fucking want to feel sad. She didn't want this feeling, and she only had it because of him, the fucking bastard. And she wanted him to know. Oh God, she wanted him to know. She could feel the sadness switch into anger, and she could feel herself tense as it increased inside her. She realised she had clenched her fists and her jaw had tightened and her teeth were firmly clamped together. 'I'll never forgive him for what he did to me. I'll never fucking forgive him. I hate him. I hate him. I fucking hate him, the bastard. He may be my father, well, he doesn't feel like one anymore, not to me. Not to me. I fucking, fucking hate him.' The volume of her voice increased.

Laura raised her voice to match Jennifer's. 'You fucking, fucking hate him.'

Jennifer knows she has been heard and that she has expressed what she feels and what part of her would like to do. This frees her up to move on to another issue.

'Part of me would like to string him up by the balls and chop it off.' Jennifer put her face in her hands, breathed in deeply and blew her breath out. 'But I know that's not the answer to anything. I also want to understand why. I don't suppose I ever will, but I'm going to talk to him again, and this time I want my mother there too, she has to answer some questions. And I need to do this before Christmas. And time is running out. I'm going back over to see them, and I need my sister to come along again if she will. I'm going to talk to her about it and just the two of us to go over this time, sort it out in the family.'

'You want to sort it out with him and your mother, sort it out within the family.'

'I've got to. I'm so much clearer on what happened now, so much more aware of it all, and there's no way I can play happy families this Christmas, no way.'

'Christmas is kind of accelerating your need to get it sorted, as well as the feelings and the clarity of what you can remember.'

'Yeah. Yeah. I'm taking that away from this session. I need to get this out in the open and somehow try and put it to rest. I just want him to admit to it, and I need to know why. And we need to make sure it doesn't happen again. And why me? Why not my sister? I don't understand that. I just don't understand that. But I'm glad that it doesn't seem to have happened to her. I'm sure that if it had, all the talking about it would have triggered something. But she doesn't remember anything. I'm glad for that. It doesn't help my memories, but perhaps his interest in me kept him away from her. I don't know. I just don't know.'

'The thought that you might have kept him away from her. So many questions, so much not knowing.'

'Yes. It can't go on like this. It's going to have repercussions, and God knows what the result will be, but he knows what he did, and so does she. I'm not protecting anyone from anything they don't already know. I want to get it out into the open, and get some answers. I know it won't take away the memories, but I know I'll feel better for it.'

'That sounds very realistic, Jennifer. How they will react, who knows. I guess you have your hopes and fears around that. But you clearly have a vivid sense that you will feel better for making it visible.'

> Laura has conveyed both acceptance and the realistic nature of what Jennifer is planning and thinking. The fact that Jennifer's sense that she will feel better whatever happens probably allows her to continue with what she sees as the worst possible scenario, and to formulate how she would deal with that as well.

'Yeah. The worst is that they'll deny it ever happened. And we'll end up shouting at each other. No, if that happens I shall just say what I need to say, what I need them to hear, and then I'll leave and it'll be up to them to respond. But I hope there will be an admission and then maybe I can get some answers and make some sense of it. And maybe we'll then know where we stand with my sister's children.' Jennifer shuddered as she said that. She suddenly became aware of how much she had been focusing on herself and suddenly remembering her niece shifted her perspective on it all. 'Yes, it's Susie, my niece, who I need to be sure about now. But I need my own answers as well.'

'Protecting Susie, but getting your own answers too?'

'Yeah.'

Laura had glanced at the clock, ten minutes left. Jennifer noticed the glance and also looked at the clock. 'I'm going to have to go to the loo, all that water I think. She got up, returning a few minutes later. 'That's better. This feels like the place to stop, Laura. Thanks, as ever. I feel like I've revealed more of me to you again, and although it did leave me feeling quite weak, I do feel stronger for it now. I don't want to go back into it. I want to go on with my thoughts about confronting my parents, and getting it sorted. And I'm glad to have got to that place. I kind of knew that I had to but I think I had been pushing it away. But today, well, I know I had to and I know it has to be sooner rather than later. I'll call my sister and see how she's fixed up. I expect she'll want to give it priority so maybe we'll, I'll, have done it by the time I see you next week. Thanks, once again.'

Counselling session 49

Jennifer was sitting in Laura's counselling room. It had just turned 7.30pm. Well, she thought to herself, it's all out in the open now. She had phoned her sister and they had agreed that it needed to be resolved ahead of Christmas. They had agreed to go to her parents that weekend, on the Saturday after she and her sister had spent Friday evening and Saturday morning together. She had made it clear to her parents that they needed to discuss some family matters.

Jennifer described all this to Laura, briefly, and then began to describe what had happened. She felt she needed to do this, in a sense to keep Laura up-to-date with developments, but she also needed her to know what had happened so she could help her explore and understand her feelings about it all, and part of her simply wanted to keep telling the story. She knew what happened when experiences got bottled up, she knew how much better she felt in herself when she expressed herself and shared her experiences, however difficult or painful they might be.

Laura sat listening to Jennifer's description of the weekend.

'So, we went over Saturday afternoon, after lunch. It somehow didn't feel right to talk about this and then sit down to lunch. I guess I got to the point very quickly, I felt I had to. I mean, it felt really difficult in one sense, but I knew things had to be said. So I told them, clearly, what I now remembered from my childhood, of my father and what he did, though I didn't go into all the graphic detail, and the fact that I knew my mother had seen it and was aware. At that point my mother burst into tears, but I needed to carry on, saying how it was affecting me and how I was trying to learn to live with the memories, but how I needed to understand why, why me, and whether he had done this to anyone else. And of course Susie, and our concerns. My sister spoke then and expressed her feelings and how she could not take any risks with her daughter, that she needed to be sure that it was not going to happen again, and how difficult it was for her to actually feel sure whatever was said.'

Laura continues listening, feeling no need to say anything other than to maintain minimal responses and acknowledgements, nodding her head, reflecting her reactions in her facial expression. Jennifer has a story she needs to tell and Laura allows her to continue without interruption.

'Well, my father started by denying it again, and getting angry, but my mother suddenly through the tears flared up at him, and screamed at him to "stop it!". She looked so sad, so so sad, she couldn't stop crying but she really did let fly at him. The anger in her face. Seemed as though years of frustrated feelings exploded out of her. I hadn't expected that, but somehow it was needed. Perhaps she was now finding her voice after so many years, I think she needed to say what she said. It was her reaction more than anything else that silenced my father. He went very pale and slumped back into his chair, his head in his hands. In fact, my mother got up and started hitting him and we had to pull her away. He didn't react. He just sat there.'

Laura nodded. 'Must have left you with so many thoughts and feelings watching this happen.'

'I'd never seen my mother like that, I mean, she had been angry with me, but I'd never seen her really lose it like that. She told him how much she had hated him, how she had tried to push the memories aside over the years and with time they seemed to have faded more and more into the background, but they had never gone away. How she had felt afraid to say anything. Then she dropped a bombshell. Told us she had been sexually abused by her father too. I hadn't expected that. I didn't know what to feel then. I wanted to say how sorry I was, but I still felt so much for myself about how she had reacted when it was happening to me.'

Laura reached over and took Jennifer's hand. Jennifer gripped her tightly.

Should Laura have made a verbal empathic response, or was a physical reaching out more appropriate?

'I've never seen my father so quiet. He just sat there, staring into space, seemed so distant, so weak somehow.' Jennifer could see him so clearly in her mind's eye. She shook her head. 'Anyway, it came out about how my mother had treated me as a poor second best to my sister, and that was because my mother felt I had been encouraging my father. Seems likely that this had grown out of her own experiences and how she had felt to blame for her father's abuse of her. You see, there was no therapy around for her in those days, she had blamed herself and carried the belief that, well, men couldn't help themselves and it was a girl's fault if it happened. I told her it was never the little girl's fault, that the adult should always be the responsible one. I was really grateful in that moment for the encouragement you had given me to realise I was not to blame. That was really important.'

Jennifer paused momentarily, and then continued. 'My mother was very tearful at that point, saying how sorry she was for how she had been. There were a lot of tears, a lot of tears, and somehow it really seemed to help clear the air. I felt closer to my mother, and I could sort of understand how her experience had left her blaming me, but at the same time I couldn't understand how, as a grown woman, she still thought that way. I guess I may never really resolve that one.'

Laura responded. 'A question you may never really resolve, how could she as your mother still carry the belief that it is the little girl's fault when she is sexually abused as she was, and as you were.' Laura knew she was experiencing some anger around this topic, it was part of the way some abusers played it, encouraging the child to blame themselves and therefore encouraging in them a sense of guilt and a greater reluctance to tell anyone for fear of being blamed.

Jennifer then told Laura how her mother was thinking of going into therapy. 'It feels like she has taken it as an opportunity. But she really did explode at my father. My God. She just went ballistic. We really did have to drag her away from him. The distress, the anger, so much must have been bottled up and she just blew.' Jennifer shook her head. 'But I'm so glad she did. So glad she was able to own and make visible those feelings.'

'Left you feeling glad for her, feeling glad about her reaction.'

'Well, it kind of felt so damned real, like she was being really and truly authentically herself. My mother has always tended to put on a kind of façade in a way, sort of keeping the peace and tending to do what she felt was expected of her, or what I guess would be in line with what others would want of her. I suppose she has been quite weak in many ways, though I never thought of it quite like that. It was just how she was. But I think things are going to change now. I don't think she is going to tolerate things quite the same, or, well, I guess compromise herself in the same way. We had a really long talk on the phone as well on Sunday and she really did sound like she was going to get a life for herself.'

'So, your mother is going to get a life for herself.'

Jennifer smiled, 'Like mother, like daughter, huh?'

'That how it feels, like mother, like daughter?'

'Yes, it does. We seem a lot closer suddenly, like a veil or a shutter has been lifted that had kept us apart somehow. I hadn't really noticed it before, just accepted that we were how we were, but now it is different and it feels good. I think it is something about our having a shared experience and being in places in ourselves in which we want to make changes, move on, I don't know, just get on with our lives but in a different way. I don't feel the distance that was obviously there between us in the past.'

'So, feeling closer, wanting to get on with your lives.' A word came to mind quite strongly as Laura said this, and it sort of echoed from her own feeling of being with Jennifer earlier in the sessions when it had felt like a real woman-to-woman experience. 'The word "solidarity" comes to my mind but that may not reflect how you experience it.'

'Yeah, that sounds good. And yet that also sounds kind of hard as well, and I'm experiencing that what we have is softer somehow. Not a weak softness, a strong softness.' Jennifer's eyes began to water as she experienced a feeling in her body and goose bumps breaking out over her arms and neck. 'I think I'm experiencing love for my mother, and I think I am experiencing her love for me.' With that she dissolved into floods of tears. Laura leaned forwards, 'Love for each other,' and paused, then continued, 'and that sounds really new and fresh.'

Laura adds this final comment about sounding really new and fresh because this is what she is sensing to be present for Jennifer, possibly a love for and from her mother that she has not experienced in a great many years, and probably not as an adult. It offers Jennifer the opportunity to recognise that sense of moving into a new experience, and this is confirmed by Jennifer's response.

'Yes. It just feels so good. Oh Laura, it's like getting my mummy back and a mother at the same time, and a good friend too. I hope it continues like this.' As she said that, Jennifer's thoughts drifted back to her father, and how he had reacted, and the uncertainty as to how he was going to be and what effect that was going to have on her and on her mother.

'I haven't said much about my father.'

'No, I was aware of that too. Did you want to say something?'

'He was really quiet, didn't really say much, in fact he made his excuses and left the room. I think he went outside. He's always found it hard to show emotion. But he did come back. I can see him coming back through the door, his head was bowed. He walked over to where I was sitting. His eyes were red. He looked at me. "I'm sorry, Jennifer, I'm so, so sorry. I can't change what happened, and I am so ashamed of what I did, and . . . ." He went silent then, and the tears were welling up in his eyes. He then said that he wanted to hug me but felt afraid to ask. I stood up and we did hug. Well, we had hugged at other times in life but somehow this felt more real, a full-on hug and we were both crying. I released myself from him and told him that I appreciated he must be feeling so many things, but that I really needed answers for myself, I needed to understand "why?", and "why me?".' He sat down next to me and told me that he didn't really understand himself. That something had come over him and he somehow felt he needed to do what he did, that it had given him pleasure but it had also given him a heavy heart as well.'

Jennifer went quiet for a moment, she was finding it very emotional to retell what had happened, feelings for her were still very present and real, and it was all very vivid in her mind.

Laura responded by acknowledging that it was OK for her to go at her own pace, and to say what she felt she needed to say.

'He said that he battled with himself, and sometimes holding me was enough, touching me was enough, but other times he just needed, wanted to do it, needed the release. He knew he had started when I was much younger, before he had spent so much time away at work, and that when he had come back he and my mother hadn't really had much of a sex life. And he didn't want to blame that, he felt that he was to blame, it was him who had come to me and made me do the things he wanted me to do to him. He said that in a way he had spent his whole life fearing that this day would come, and at the same time pushing it aside and denying to himself it had ever happened. Sometimes he had felt that it really had all been some crazy dream. At other times the memories were more real. He was ashamed and he didn't know what to say or do.'

'So he expressed being ashamed and blamed himself. How was that? Was that enough for you?'

'No.' Jennifer's response came back fast. 'No it wasn't. I told him what about when I was younger, three, four, whenever it started, sitting on his lap, and how he even tried to penetrate me then. I hadn't actually mentioned that before. At that moment my mother broke down. She genuinely hadn't realised that that had been happening. Oh God, it was horrible, it was an awful time. I was upset, my mother was crying pitifully and cursing my father. He was lost, didn't know what to say or do. Thank God my sister was there. She comforted my mother and in fact suggested that the two of them go out for a walk and leave me and my father to carry on talking. That was probably the best thing that could have happened. We needed that time.'

'So your mother and sister left for a while, and you carried on talking with your father.' Laura again kept her response brief to allow Jennifer to continue with her narrative.

'At first we sat in silence. Then he broke the silence by saying that he did not know what to do, that he heard my need for answers but he was struggling to find them, that he had tried to find them for himself and hadn't been able to make sense of it, at least not at the start when I was really young. Yes, he knew he had an attraction towards young girls, that yes, it did arouse him, or at least it used to, but it had stopped a long time ago.'

Laura nodded, holding her heart open to Jennifer, maintaining her unconditional warmth for her as she continued.

'I asked if there were others. He hesitated and said no. I challenged his hesitation. He cried at that, and told me that when he had been overseas there had been young girls available, and he had at times been with some. He felt that had probably left him feeling it was acceptable somehow, and that somehow he had made himself feel it was acceptable to do it with me. But he had no answer to when I was younger. That, he said, is something "I will never understand and will have to carry with me for the rest of my life". I told him he wasn't the only one, and we both went quiet for a while.'

'I asked about my sister and he said no, and again he couldn't explain why, other than he had me and that was enough for him. That he kind of felt that my sister was too close to my mother, and he feared she would tell. He didn't know that my mother was aware of what was happening and was saying nothing.' She stopped for a moment then continued. 'It's very fragile between my father and mother now, and I'm not sure what I feel anymore towards my father. Pity is there – that only emerged out of the weekend. I'm relieved that he owned up to it, but he still did it. And I'll never forget that, and not just me, those girls when he was overseas. I feel sick thinking about it.'

'So you pity him, have no respect and feel sick at the thought of all the other girls when he was overseas.' Laura could see a look in Jennifer's face that to her expressed revulsion. She empathised with that as well. 'The look on your face seems to me to be one of utter revulsion.'

Hearing it said back to her really gave Jennifer time and focus to be with her feelings more deeply. She realised how much she despised her father. She didn't know if it was going to be a phase or a permanent attitude, but it was where she was in the present. She sat with her feelings for a moment.

A simple empathic response has offered Jennifer the opportunity to simply be with her feelings. It has given her a break from talking about what happened and about the effect on her. It created a space for her to simply be with the feelings and be affected by them in the present and in the context of the therapeutic relationship with Laura. It can be, and often is, a very powerful experience for the client. The therapeutic value of empathy should never be underestimated.

'I need these feelings at the moment, Laura, and I know they are hurtful to my father in particular, but I do need to feel what I feel. It is part of me, of who I am, and I have to claim myself in all of this. I don't know what I am going to do with what I feel, I really don't, and I know long term I don't want to lose touch with my father, but I know that at the moment I need distance from him and time to be with what is . . . ,' she took a deep breath and let it out forcefully, 'be with what is going on inside me.'

'Those feelings are important to you, they are part of you, you want to be with them, whatever the effect on your family.'

'That sounds hard, hearing you say it, and yet that's how it is. That's how it is.' Jennifer lifted her hands to her face, rubbed her eyes with her fingertips and breathed deeply again. She took her hands away. 'I'm going to survive all this. It feels like a nightmare, and it is a nightmare, but I am going to survive. I know it is going to take time, and many more hours of talking to you, and finding my own ways of making sense of it all. But I am so grateful to you, Laura, for being there, being here. I had no idea back in May that all of this was going to blow up, there I was thinking my therapy was coming to a close, and yet within me a storm was gathering, and I had no idea. Part of me wishes none of it had surfaced, but I know now that it had to, and maybe it has happened at the right time, a time when I can deal with it. I know the drinking got problematic again, and I still haven't completely reigned that back in, but if all this had come to the surface a few years back, when the alcohol and cocaine were really dominating my life . . . .' Jennifer shook her head and spoke softly. 'I don't think I would still be here.'

Laura nodded. 'That bad?'

'Yeah, I'd have fallen apart and used whatever drugs were around. I'd have gone for the quick anaesthetic fix.' She again lifted her hands to her face and blew out a breath. 'Part of me feels lucky to be here. And I have a future to look forward to. God knows, Ian has ridden the storm with me these last few months, he has been so rock solid, so sensitive, so caring towards me. He must love me so much. I don't want to lose that now. And I do want a family, and will have one. We are working on it!' She smiled at that and Laura smiled back.

'Ian has been so important, hasn't he?'

'Unbelievably so, and you, in a different way of course. And my sister, particularly for not doubting me. None of you doubted me, even when I was doubting myself.'

'I accept you and what is real to you, Jennifer, and I always want to be open to anything and everything that you bring to these sessions. The impact on me of what has happened in recent months has been huge, and it has all felt so very,

very real. At times it felt like you were gathering pieces of a jigsaw and trying to work out how they fitted, and gradually a picture emerged, but not a very nice picture. A painful, harrowing and deeply disturbing one.'

Jennifer picked up on the metaphor. 'And I still only have some of the pieces in place, but they have been enough to get me to where I am today, and it feels like there are more pieces to find and, with your help, I hope I can piece them together, and maybe then I'll be able to break it all up and put it away. I feel that's what I will need to do, but I am not there yet. I'm sure the coming months will be, what can I say, difficult? Sounds a silly word. I'm growing, Laura, and I'm going to grow through and out of all this. And I don't know what I will be like, and that doesn't matter. I just wish the hurt would go away, but then, that would be impossible. What happened, happened, and I have to come to terms with it and learn to manage reactions that I have that were established in the past.'

Jennifer commented that time was nearly up, and the session, but not the process, drew to a close.

The process would continue over many more sessions, bringing a whole range of experiences. Some would be positive and celebratory of growth and achievement, of change and transition into the person, the woman, that Jennifer would become. Others would be painful and challenging, pitching Jennifer back into aspects of herself that left her feeling sad, self-doubting and questioning whether it was all worth it. But the process was running. Jennifer was receiving a regular experience of those core conditions of empathy, unconditional positive regard and congruence that are so fundamental to positive therapeutic change. Of these, Rogers wrote, 'in our work as person-centred therapists and facilitators, we have discovered the attitudinal qualities that are demonstrably effective in releasing constructive and growthful changes in the personality and behaviour of individuals. Persons in an environment infused with these attitudes develop more self-understanding, more self-confidence, more ability to choose their behaviours. They learn more significantly, they have more freedom to be and become' (Rogers, 1980, p. 133).

As Jennifer left, Laura noted that she felt a big hurdle had been crossed. Jennifer's past was now visible and the family system had been confronted and forced into reality and authenticity. Whether the glue, the love, would prove strong enough to hold it together was for the future to decide. But at least the truth was out and everyone could now begin to come to terms with it more openly. Yes, it had caused intense pain – these kinds of experiences inevitably do. But Laura felt that Jennifer could now get on with her own process of redefining herself in a way that was increasingly free of her past conditioning. She, Laura, felt good to be part of that process and she looked forward to the future sessions and the continuing development of their therapeutic relationship.

Then a final thought struck her, something that Jennifer had not actually mentioned having raised and discussed with her father. Was Susie, Jennifer's niece, really going to be safe?

Points for discussion

- Had Laura intervened and suggested a more cautionary approach to Jennifer regarding her decision to go for her enhanced role at work, what might have been the effect on Jennifer?
- Do you feel that you can trust your client's process? What might make it difficult for you to experience this trust, and why? How would you resolve this?
- The idea of shared silence within the counselling session. How would you summarise the value in this?
- Should Laura have reflected back the phrases that Jennifer's father had used when he had come into the room? Would it have had therapeutic value to have done so?
- How would you evaluate the overall quality of Laura's empathy during these sessions?
- What reactions did you experience as you read these sessions, and what impact would they have had on you had you been Jennifer's counsellor?
- What other kinds of reaction might have occurred from Jennifer's family, and what effect might this have had?
- The sessions will continue. What issues do you anticipate will need to be addressed? List them and reflect on how they might be therapeutically resolved in the context of person-centred working.

CHAPTER 9

Jennifer reflects on her experience as a client

I really thought that the counselling was coming to an end early in the summer. I felt good. I felt I had resolved so many issues and was feeling positive about my life. I couldn't believe what then emerged. Hearing myself speaking in that session when I talked about what had happened to me when I was about four, oh God, that was an awful shock. It was so real, so horribly real. And from then on it just got worse. And all, seemingly, triggered by that look, that expression I saw on my father's face when he had Susie on his lap.

I seem to have been put through an emotional mangle these past few months, so many feelings have been squeezed out of me, and memories that I had no idea I carried. I have had to face up to experiences that I never dreamed of as being part of my past. But the dreams were all too real.

I feel so incredibly indebted to Laura. She was so steady. It probably helped that we had already spent about 11 months meeting, and perhaps the fact that I felt so at ease with her made it easier for me to bring my experiences to her. At the same time, I wonder whether I really had any choice in the matter. The flashbacks that occurred in the sessions, the hearing parts of myself as voices echoing from the past, and slipping out-of-body, I had no control over them. But at least Laura stayed with me. She didn't seem fazed by any of it, though I am sure she bent her supervisor's ear on more than one occasion. I know I had a profound effect on her. I saw it in her facial expression on a number of occasions, and particularly in her eyes. Probably when I saw the tears in her eyes was one of the most powerful experiences for me, it really validated what I was experiencing at the time, somehow it helped something change within me. And I am so glad Laura allowed me to see, feel and be touched by her humanity. But that wasn't the only occasion.

Another moment that stands out was when she came over and hugged me, held me, in that moment when I just felt I needed a mother like Laura. That just triggered such a release for me, but more than that, a real confirmation somehow that I was lovable. I hadn't registered that at the time and it is only now, in hindsight, that I can see the power of that moment. Funny, isn't it, with all the talking and listening, the two moments that stand out were non-verbal. Yet alone they could not have been enough. The verbal content was so necessary, 'part of the process', as I am sure Laura would say.

Whatever happened, however I was with her, she stayed with me, she kept listening, she kept taking me seriously, she kept caring. More than anything else, these are the things that meant so much during those sessions.

Where I work I often hear people rubbishing therapy, not that most of them have had any experience. I tend not to get drawn in, but occasionally I have. I try to point out that I can only speak from my own experience, that I have found it extremely helpful. When they ask what was helpful, I tell them that it is simple, though I am sure it is not that simple for the counsellor. I tell them that for me the most powerful thing was to feel listened to and to be taken seriously. That to be with someone who didn't tell you what to think or how to feel was liberating, that it has liberated me from parts of me, and liberated me to become more of who I am. Their eyes often glaze over at that bit. But I tell them that it has helped me make sense of myself and to learn to make choices and decisions that are genuinely right for me, and based on my own sense of what my needs are. I tell them they should try it if they really want to know what it is about.

I felt loved in those therapy sessions, and I still do as the process continues. It's a word we often shy away from, but it is what I experienced. Some people may call it warmth, or I believe the technical term is unconditional positive regard, but for me it was about feeling loved, as a person, as a woman, as Jennifer. At times we felt very close, and it felt spiritual, not in some religious sense, but in feeling a deep connection with Laura and with myself. When such moments occurred I felt the stronger for it. I felt I grew out of them, moved forwards in some way even though I may not have been able to define in words exactly what had happened.

I know I still have much more work to do on myself. But now I can see a little more clearly. I have faced the demon inside me and I am still alive and breathing. I am sure aspects of it will continue to rise up at me, but now I must persevere in rebuilding my life. I think that the trick in therapy is not only to focus on breaking down the old, the negative conditioning, but it must also involve building the new. I needed to look back, and at times I still do, but increasingly I am looking ahead, but from a greater sense of security within myself as I stand in the present.

Sometimes I can't believe what happened to me. But that doubt is just a trick of the light. It happened. And I am learning to move on. Life after sexual abuse. On good days I can breathe that life in and it feels like oxygen. It enriches and nourishes me. I am finding new ways of looking after myself. I have become more conscious of exercise, healthy eating, not overdoing it and getting stressed out. I can appreciate my body again. I don't have to only think of it as dirty or unclean as I once did.

Oh, and I'm pregnant, must have happened around the session when I experienced that sense of OKness. Guess I relaxed a little more and the time was right. I don't know if it will be a boy or a girl, I really don't mind, at least, I don't think I mind. Maybe I'd like a little girl. I think I might have been afraid to say that at one time, I would have feared for her. But now? Now I know what it can be like to feel free, and I want her to have that experience. So maybe I do want a little girl after all.

I want to end by returning back to the theme of my counselling. I want to say that if you are troubled by disturbing memories, dreams, behaviours that just don't feel right somehow, think about talking it over with a therapist, and I would recommend a person-centred one, but you may find someone with a different approach. At the end of the day, I'm not sure whether it is the approach or the person that matters most. But make sure they are a good listener, they ring true and authentic, and they convey the sense of genuinely caring about you as a person.

Laura reviews the counselling process from her perspective

Always expect the unexpected. You only know as much as a client discloses. They may hold back, they may simply not be fully aware of experiences that have affected them. Make no assumptions, take nothing for granted, be open to possibilities. Of course I knew all this, but my encounter with Jennifer taught me the truth of all of them. I had no idea what was going to emerge. It goes to show once again that Rogers was right in saying that the client's process has to be trusted. What emerged did so when the time was right for Jennifer to deal with it. And I felt privileged to be part of that, and still do as our work continues.

Like so many who have had to face up to the reality of being the target of child sexual abuse – and yes, the child is always the victim, let's be clear about that – Jennifer had to face herself and her family. And she has done, and continues to do, this. She is learning to move from target to survivor. And her family must also now tread that same path, and to survive what has been made visible to all.

I have been deeply affected by Jennifer, by her experiences, by the intensity of her presence, by her openness to being who she is within the counselling sessions. The discussion in that last session about finding pieces of a jigsaw really did sum up for me how I was experiencing it, although somehow pieces of a jigsaw are a bit set and fixed, and I see it as perhaps a little more fluid than that. However, the metaphor is apt. People come into counselling often not even being aware of the bag of jigsaw pieces they carry with them, or they are aware of a few, or what they have they have assembled as best they can, although more often than not the pieces they have are largely those given to them by others through their reactions to the client, particularly but not exclusively in early life. Parts of the picture come together and, as with Jennifer, can reveal a shocking reality. So often time has to be spent building parts of the picture before starting to let go of some of the pieces, and beginning to create and assemble new pieces.

Jennifer was at first unaware of some of the pieces she brought, but gradually they began to demand attention. Her 4-year-old self spoke and drew her, and my attention, to distressing facts from her past. Later, through dreams and flashbacks, other pieces revealed themselves. She doubted what she saw, but was able to acknowledge it's truth. I think the acceptance of her that I sought to convey helped and, I think crucially, so did the reaction of her sister. A disturbing picture emerged. Unsettling. She could have tried to break it up and hide it away in a box, but she was brave enough not to do that. She was tempted, the alcohol use increased, often a favourite way of blotting out that which is unsettling. But she brought that largely under control and brought the picture to the attention of her partner, her sister and then her parents. An act of great courage.

I sought to keep in touch with what Jennifer told me and described about her inner world, and often I found myself not saying very much, but rather allowing Jennifer to do the work for herself. It seemed at times that I was more of a facilitator than a counsellor, facilitating Jennifer's own growth process, or at least trying to avoid getting in the way of it! I think I managed that, although there were times when my own feelings and assumptions did get into the dialogue. But then, I think that the person-centred counsellor is very much a facilitator. He or she recognises that within the client is a tendency towards growth or constructive personality change, and that if the right conditions can be made available that tendency will encourage the client towards increasingly fulfilling and satisfying experiences, behaviours and choices. Trust in that actualising tendency is crucial.

I don't think I tried to make anything happen for Jennifer, or to make her see things a certain way, or take a particular direction. I hope not, anyway. I wanted her to find – or is it make – her own path. There were so many silences, and I do respect silence as such a powerful experience, and potentially so therapeutic. And she was so fragile at times, strongly affected by the feelings associated with her regained memories. I was concerned that her alcohol use might really get out of control, and she might also go back to other substances to quell the emotional battering she was receiving. But I did not go on about those concerns in the sessions. I could have simply amplified an unease that may have been present for her and made it worse. I trusted her ability to make the choices she needed to make, and that included what she wanted to bring to the sessions.

I so wanted to listen, to hear, what Jennifer wanted to tell me, what was present for her in those sessions. I feel passionately about the importance of person-to-person encounter. I wanted to meet Jennifer, to breathe her world, and at times I felt that I did. I hope that she felt this passion within me, and the caring I felt for her as a woman, and particularly as a woman fighting back against one of the most undermining and invasive experiences that a person can have. And then to discover that her mother had gone through the same ordeal, but had been left with a very different experience, carrying the memory throughout her life and the belief that she had been to blame. When I had first heard how her mother had watched without taking action I had gone cold. I'm still not sure now that there was really an excuse for that lack of response, but at least I appreciate the why, and so does Jennifer. But the why question has not been answered by her father to Jennifer's satisfaction and it is unlikely that it ever will.

There is more work to do, the healing process takes time. Part of this is likely to involve further engagement with her anger (which Bass and Davis (1988) refer to as 'the backbone of healing'). She may also want to learn ways to control going out-of-body, if that is what she wishes for. She also has the experience of pregnancy now which is likely to trigger experiencing linked to her traumatised past, and throughout which she will need deep emotional support.

So, the sessions continue, and gradually I see Jennifer changing and freeing herself from her past, not to forget, but to find ways of recreating herself in such a way that she can carry the memories but let go of the conditioning effects. Of course, the emotional scars will probably never go away. But I feel confident that she will grow through all of this, and I genuinely look forward to each session, whatever the content. There is something deeply satisfying about being in a healing relationship that is growing towards greater and fuller authenticity.

Some final thoughts

This book does not reflect the whole process, but rather a period within which childhood memories of sexual abuse have started to come into conscious awareness and the effect that this has. This can take place over a relatively short period of time, or much longer. The length of therapy then needed to fully deal with what emerges will vary from person to person, but a minimum of a year from the time of remembering can be anticipated, and generally it is more.

So what you have read may feel a little condensed, intensifying the effect on the reader. I make no apology for this. My aim all along has been to make an impact, to stir up feelings and to trigger thoughts and reflection.

How Jennifer will grow in the future is unknown. She is a person in her own right and will take directions in her life that will satisfy and fulfil her needs as she experiences them. No one can say for sure what form this will actually take. So no goals can be set for her to aim for other than those that she sets for herself. She knows what she wants to achieve, and this may change, and probably will, as time goes by.

I hope that this book has opened your heart and your mind to something of the process of counselling a survivor of child sexual abuse from a person-centred perspective. It is a rewarding area of work. One of the most powerful experiences we can have as human beings is to witness a person claiming their personhood, increasingly free of the conditioning of the past, and associated traumatic memories. More powerful still is to play a part in facilitating that process through the creation of a warm, respectful, authentic and empathic relationship with another person who is in pain. As person-centred counsellors, or whatever your role may be in helping people through the trauma of child sexual abuse, work at creating right and respectful relationships with your clients.

I can do no better than end with a quote from Peggy Natiello, a person-centred therapist and group facilitator, who I know has been an inspiration to many, including myself.

'Healing in therapy is in direct proportion to the quality of the relationship' (Natiello, 2001, p. 28).

References

Armstrong L (1978) *Kiss Daddy Goodnight: a speak-out on incest.* Pocket Books, New York.

Bagley C and King K (1990) *Child Sexual Abuse: the search for healing.* Routledge, London.

Bass E and Davis L (1988) *The Courage to Heal: a guide for woman survivors of child sexual abuse.* Harper and Row, New York, and Vermilion, London (1997).

Bass E and Davis L (1991) *Allies in Healing.* Perennial Library, Harper and Row, New York.

Bass E and Davis L (1993) *Beginning to Heal: the first guide for female survivors of child sexual abuse.* Cedar, London.

Bonaparte M, Freud A and Kris E (eds) (1954) *The Origins of Psychoanalysis: letters to Wilhem Fliess, drafts and notes by Sigmund Freud* (Basic Books, New York, pp. 215–6). Referred to in Herman JL (1992) *Trauma and Recovery.* Basic Books, New York.

Bozarth J (1998) *Person-Centred Therapy: a revolutionary paradigm.* PCCS Books, Ross-on-Wye.

Bozarth J and Wilkins P (eds) (2001) *Rogers' Therapeutic Conditions: evolution, theory and practice.* Volume 3. *Unconditional Positive Regard.* PCCS Books, Ross-on-Wye.

Bryant-Jefferies R (2001) *Counselling the Person Beyond the Alcohol Problem.* Jessica Kingsley Publishers, London.

Bryant-Jefferies R (2003) *Problem Drinking: a person-centred dialogue.* Radcliffe Medical Press, Oxford.

Davis L (1990) *The Courage to Heal Workbook: for women and men survivors of child sexual abuse.* Perennial Library, Harper and Row, New York.

Draucker CB (1992) *Counselling Survivors of Childhood Sexual Abuse.* Sage, London.

Freud S (1896) The aetiology of hysteria. In: *Standard Edition*, volume 3, trans. Strachey J (1962) Hogarth Press, London, p. 203. Quoted in Herman JL (1992) *Trauma and Recovery.* Basic Books, New York.

Gaylin N (2001) *Family, Self and Psychotherapy: a person-centred perspective.* PCCS Books, Ross-on-Wye.

Goldstein AP (1980) Relationship enhancement methods. In: FH Kanfer and AP Goldstein (eds) *Helping People Change: a textbook of methods* (2e). Pergamon, New York.

Haugh S and Merry T (eds) (2001) *Rogers' Therapeutic Conditions: evolution, theory and practice.* Volume 2: *Empathy.* PCCS Books, Ross-on-Wye.

Herman JL (1994) *Trauma and Recovery*. Pandora, London. Originally published by Basic Books, New York.

Herman JL and Schatzow E (1987) Recovery and verification of memories of childhood sexual trauma. *Psychoanalytic Psychology*. 4: 1–14.

Kepner JL (1995) *Healing Tasks: psychotherapy with adult survivors of childhood abuse*. Jossey Bass Publishers, San Francisco.

Kinsey AC, Pomeroy WB, Martin CE and Gebbard PH (1953) *Sexual Behaviour in the Human Female*. Saunders, Philadelphia.

Mearns D and Thorne B (1988) *Person-Centred Counselling in Action*. Sage, London.

Mearns D and Thorne B (1999) *Person-Centred Counselling in Action* (2e). Sage, London.

Merry T (1999) *Learning and Being in Person-Centred Counselling*. PCCS Books, Ross-on-Wye.

Natiello P (2001) *The Person-Centred Approach: a passionate presence*. PCCS Books, Ross-on-Wye.

Peters SD, Wyatt GE and Finkelhor D (1986) Prevalence. In: D Findelhor (ed.) *A Source Book of Child Sexual Abuse*. Sage, Beverley Hills, CA, pp. 15–59.

Rogers CR (1957) The necessary and sufficient conditions of therapeutic personality change. *Journal of Consulting Psychology*. 21: 95–103.

Rogers CR (1959) The way to do is to be. *American Psychologist*. 4: 197. Quoted in: P Natiello (2001) *The Person-Centred Approach: a passionate presence*. PCCS Books, Ross-on-Wye.

Rogers CR (1980) *A Way of Being*. Houghton-Mifflin Company, Boston, MA.

Russell DEH (1983) The incidence and prevalence of inter-familial and extra-familial sexual assault of female children. *Child Abuse and Neglect*. 7: 133–46.

Russell DEH (1986) *The Secret Trauma: incest in the lives of girls and women*. Basic Books, New York.

Sanderson C (1990) *Counselling Adult Survivors of Child Sexual Abuse*. Jessica Kingsley Publishers, London.

Sanderson C (1995) *Counselling Adult Survivors of Child Sexual Abuse* (2e). Jessica Kingsley Publishers, London.

Spak L, Spak F and Allebeck P (1997) Factors in childhood and youth predicting alcohol dependence and abuse in Swedish women: findings from a general population study. *Alcohol and Alcoholism*. 32: 267–74.

Swett Jr C, Cohen C, Surrey J *et al.* (1991) High rates of alcohol use and history of physical and sexual abuse among women outpatients. *American Journal of Drug Alcohol Abuse*. 17(1): 49–60.

Taylor SE (1983) Adjustment to threatening events: a theory of cognitive adaptation. *American Psychologist*. 38: 1161–73.

Warner MS (1998) A client-centered approach to therapeutic work with dissociated and fragile process. In: L Greenberg, J Watson and G Lietaer (eds) *Handbook of Experiential Psychotherapy*. The Guildford Press, New York, pp. 368–87.

Warner MS and Mearns D (2000) *Multiple Configurations of Self in Client-Centered Therapy*. Joint paper presented to the Fifth International Conference in Client-Centered and Experiential Psychotherapy, Chicago, June.

Warner M (2000) Person-centred therapy at the difficult edge: a developmentally based model of fragile and dissociated process. In: D Mearns and B Thorne (eds) *Person-Centred Therapy Today*. Sage Publications, London.

Warner M (2002) Psychological contact, meaningful process and human nature. In: G Wyatt and P Sanders (eds) *Rogers' Therapeutic Conditions: evolution, theory and practice*. Volume 4: *Contact and Perception*. PCCS Books, Ross on Wye, pp. 76–95.

Williams DJ (1992) Supervision: a new word is desperately needed. In: S Palmer, S Dainow and P Milner (eds) *Counselling, The BAC Counselling Reader*. Sage, London.

Wyatt G (2001) *Rogers' Therapeutic Conditions: evolution, theory and practice*. Volume 1: *Congruence*. PCCS Books, Ross-on-Wye.

Wyatt G and Saunders P (2002) *Rogers' Therapeutic Conditions: evolution, theory and practice*. Volume 4: *Contact and Perception*. PCCS Books, Ross-on-Wye.

Further reading

Bryant-Jefferies R (2003) *Time Limited Therapy in Primary Care: a person-centred dialogue*. Radcliffe Medical Press, Oxford.

O'Leary C (1999) *Counselling Couples and Families: a person-centred approach*. Sage Publications, London.

Merry T (2001) Congruence and the supervision of client-centred therapists. In: G Wyatt (ed.) *Rogers' Therapeutic Conditions: evolution, theory and practice*. Volume 1: *Congruence*. PCCS Books, Ross-on-Wye.

Rogers CR (1986) A client-centered/person-centered approach to therapy. In: I Kutash and A Wolf (eds) *Psychotherapists' Casebook*. Jossey Bass, San Francisco, pp. 236–57.

Simon D (1998) *Guiding Recovery from Child Sexual Abuse: horizons of hope*. Jessica Kingsley Publishers, London.

Useful contacts

Directory and Book Services (DABS) National Resource Directory: Overcoming Childhood Sexual Abuse
1 Broxholme Lane
Doncaster
South Yorkshire DN1 2LJ
Tel: 01302 768689
Email: info@dabsbooks.co.uk
Website: www.dabsbooks.co.uk
A Directory listing over 500 services in England, Scotland and Wales working for recovery from childhood sexual abuse. Also provides a confidential mail order book service for survivors of childhood sexual abuse.

BASPCAN (British Association for the Study and Prevention of Child Abuse and Neglect)
10 Priory Street
York YO1 6EZ
Tel: 01904 613605
Email: baspcan@baspcan.org.uk
Website: www.baspcan.org.uk
A multi-disciplinary networking association for professionals working in the field of prevention and recovery from child abuse. They produce a journal, *Child Abuse Review*, and a newsletter.

Breaking Free
Suite 21–25
Marshall House
124 Middleton Road
Morden
Surrey SM4 6RW
Helpline: 020 8648 3500
A registered charity providing a safe, confidential, supportive, understanding and non-judgemental environment for women to deal with issues arising from their experiences of sexual abuse as children. It offers a national telephone helpline and support by letter, and produces a quarterly newsletter.

British Association for Counselling and Psychotherapy (BACP)
1 Regent Place
Rugby
Warwickshire CV21 2PJ
Tel: 0870 443 5252
Email: bacp@bacp.co.uk
Website: www.bacp.co.uk
National association that can provide lists of individual counsellors, psycho-therapists and professional bodies offering therapy. Also produces the British Association for Counselling and Psychotherapy Resources Directory.

Careline
The Cardinal Heenan Centre
326–328 High Road
Ilford
Essex IG1 1QP
Helpline: 020 8514 1177
National confidential crisis telephone counselling service for children, young people and adults.

Children 1st
41 Polworth Terrace
Edinburgh EH11 1NU
Helpline: 0808 800 2222
Email: info@children1st.org.uk
Website: www.children1st.org.uk
Supports families under stress; protects children from harm and neglect; helps children recover from abuse and promotes children's rights and interests. Help-line for parents and carers. Provides regional projects.

Fire in Ice
88 Rodney Street
Liverpool L1 9AR
Helpline: 0151 707 2614
Email: fireinice@freenet.co.uk
Website: www.fireinice.co.uk
A self-help project run by and for adult male survivors of childhood abuse, espe-cially those who suffered whilst in residential care.

International Association for the Study of Dissociation
60 Revere Drive
Suite 500
Northbrook
IL 60062
USA
Email: info@issd.org
Website: www.issd.org

The International Society for the Study of Dissociation is a non-profit association organised for the purposes of: information sharing and international networking of clinicians and researchers; providing professional and public education; promoting research and theory about dissociation; and promoting research and training in the identification, treatment, and prevention of dissociative disorders.

MOSAC – Supporting Non-Abusing Parents/Carers of Sexually Abused Children
London Borough of Greenwich
Helpline: 0800 980 1958
Website: www.mosac.org.uk
National helpline for parents and carers of children who have been sexually abused. Counselling, art therapy and befriending available together with group support.

Survivors UK
PO Box 2470
London SW9 6WQ
Helpline: 020 7357 6677
Email: info@survivorsuk.org.uk
Website: www.survivorsuk.org.uk
National helpline offering information, support and counselling to anyone affected by the sexual assault of men. One-to-one counselling and support groups for male survivors in the London area.

The Foundation for the Developing Person
Website: www.thefdp.demon.co.uk
Training organisation for working with survivors of childhood abuse.

Person-centred

British Association for the Person-Centred Approach (BAPCA)
Bm-BAPCA
London WC1N 3XX
Tel: 01989 770948
Email: info@bapca.org.uk
Website: www.bapca.org.uk
National association promoting the person-centred approach. Publishes the journal *Person-centred Practice* and a regular newsletter, *Person-to-Person*.

World Association for Person-Centered and Experiential Psychotherapy and Counselling
Email: secretariat@pce-world.org
Website: www.pce-world.org

Association for the Development of the Person-Centered Approach (ADPCA)
Email: adpca-web@signs.portents.com
Website: www.adpca.org
An international association, with members in 27 countries, for those interested
in the development of client-centred therapy and the person-centred approach.

Person-Centred Therapy Scotland
Tel: 0870 7650871
Email: info@pctscotland.co.uk
Website: www.pctscotland.co.uk
An association of person-centred therapists in Scotland which offers training and
networking opportunities to members with the aim of fostering high standards of
professional practice.

Index